Foreword

Health care is expensive, and resources are constrained. Doctors and health care managers throughout the world have a responsibility to spend their Treasuries' or insurers' monies on care that is effective in achieving defined successful outcomes. It is hoped that the withdrawal from ineffective care will release resources for more effective care.

Patients and their doctors usually share similar perspectives on what is effective, but this is not always so. For example, the technical benefits of physiotherapy in improving function after a stroke are not easy to measure or to distinguish from spontaneous recovery, but stroke patients feel empowered and supported by the multi-disciplinary efforts to aid them. This sense of empowerment is surely an outcome that must be considered just as much as an improvement in gait.

Health professionals are concerned to do their best for the patients under their care, and health service managers have a responsibility to ensure that the care in their locality matches the best in the country. There is therefore increasing interest in comparative measures of outcome between different teams and different localities. There are, however, enormous problems of measurement. Not only must there be suitable adjustments for severity of disease and other accompanying illnesses (co-morbidity), but the properties of any measurement instrument, such as the validity, inter-rater reliability, sensitivity to change, time-dependancy and cost of collection must also be considered.

The editors of this book determined to explore some of these issues head-on; not in relation to what might be considered the easier task of an acute event such as myocardial infarction, but rather in relation to a highly variable and often chronic illness: rheumatoid arthritis. I believe this book will be of interest not only to those concerned with helping patients with rheumatological disorders, but also to many others who will find it an illuminating illustration of the discipline of outcomes measurement.

July 1996   ANTHONY HOPKINS
                        Director, Research Unit, Royal College of Physicians

Contributors

Jean Ashcroft *Director of Policy and Campaigning, Arthritis Care, 18 Stephenson Way, London NW1 2HD*

Alison Brettle *Information Officer, UK Clearing House on Health Outcomes, Nuffield Institute for Health, University of Leeds, 71–75 Clarendon Road, Leeds LS2 9PL*

Alison J Carr *Research Associate, Department of Social Medicine, University of Bristol, Canyage Hall, Whiteladies Road, Bristol BS8 1TH*

Roy Carr-Hill *Senior Research Fellow, Centre for Health Economics, University of York, York YO1 5DD*

Paul Dixon *Senior Research Fellow, UK Clearing House on Health Outcomes, Nuffield Institute for Health, University of Leeds, 71–75 Clarendon Road, Leeds LS2 9PL*

David V Doyle *Consultant Rheumatologist, Whipps Cross Hospital, Whipps Cross Road, London E11 1NR*

Ray Fitzpatrick *Fellow of Nuffield College and University Lecturer, Department of Public Health and Primary Care, University of Oxford, Oxford OX1 1NF*

Andrew F Long *Project Leader, UK Clearing House on Health Outcomes, Nuffield Institute for Health, University of Leeds, 71–75 Clarendon Road, Leeds LS2 9PL*

David L Scott *Reader in Rheumatology, Department of Clinical and Academic Rheumatology, King's College Hospital, Denmark Hill, London SE5 9RS*

Deborah P M Symmons *Consultant Senior Lecturer, ARC Epidemiology Research Unit, School of Epidemiology and Health Sciences, Stopford Building, University of Manchester, Oxford Road, Manchester M13 9PT*

Contents

1 | Exploring outcomes: approaches and key issues

Andrew F Long
Project Leader, UK Clearing House for Health Outcomes,
Nuffield Institute for Health, University of Leeds

Introduction

Outcomes have achieved a high profile in policy discussions. The development of the internal market and commissioning process and the emphasis on health gain within the health strategy (Department of Health 1992) have pushed the assessment of health services outcomes to the centre stage of the NHS. There is an increasing emphasis on identifying what works (the effectiveness of interventions) with the intention of optimising outcomes within the context of available resources. There is thus a need for systematic evidence on effectiveness and the clarification of desired and achieved outcomes of health care interventions or episodes of care. Some of the key issues on the outcomes agenda are summarised in Table 1.

Assessing the effectiveness and outcomes of an intervention is not straightforward. To assess effectiveness necessarily involves assessing the outcomes of the intervention. But there may be a

Table 1. Issues on the outcome agenda

- Clarifying the desired outcomes of an intervention or package of care
- Identifying which interventions or packages of care work/produce these outcomes, based on available (best) research evidence
- Exploring whether the interventions or packages of care work within this setting; that is, what are the achieved outcomes within routine practice?
- Uncovering how the interventions or packages of care can be provided such that they are done better
- Establishing an outcomes management system through, for example, the use of clinical audit to use information from monitoring achieved outcomes to achieve better outcomes

variety of outcome criteria and differing perspectives on the part of the health care professional and the patient and/or carer over what an appropriate outcome may be. There is also the key issue of attribution—was the observed outcome brought about by the intervention itself or something else—and timescale over which to assess outcome.

Health commissioning agencies want to know what works, with whom and where, and to have information on outcomes achieved by service providers. Health care providers need to know whether the outcome of treatment is beneficial and to ensure high quality service provision. At the level of the individual health care practitioner—clinician, nurse and therapy professions—outcome measurement is an integral part of routine clinical practice, exploring the desired outcomes of their patients, monitoring their progress, and deciding the next stage of their treatment or care. Outcomes data are also desired by health care consumers, informing them of treatment options and consequences, and involving them in treatment decisions.

Defining outcome

Outcomes are the results (effects) of processes. They are that part of the output of a process which can be attributed to the process. Against this simple definition, three issues arise. First, to assess outcomes, inputs must be measured, including patient characteristics; accurate descriptions and assessments of process elements made; and other (confounding) factors which might have brought about any observed change, or lack of change, must be controlled for (Table 2). In other words, there must be strong grounds for suspicion that the process may lead to the outcome. Second, different actors involved in the provision of the intervention (for example, the user, the carer, the GP, the purchaser, the providing clinical team) will have different interests and potentially different desired outcomes and thus measures of outcome. Third, there is the question of timescale—is focus lying on short-term (at the end of this particular episode of care) or longer-term consequences?

An approach to assessing outcome

At the UK Clearing House on Health Outcomes in Leeds (Long 1995) a step-by-step framework has been developed to assist purchasers and providers in monitoring and assessing health outcomes and in using effectiveness evidence within clinical practice

Table 2. Requirements for health outcome measurement

- Health to be defined and monitored over time
- The effects on health are linked to the process concerned, thus the effects are shown to be 'outcomes' and not just a different state of health
- Any mediating factors are defined

  Process → Mediating factors → Outcome

(Table 3). The starting point is to clarify and identify the desired outcomes and outcome objectives of the various actors involved—at a minimum, users, carers and the multidisciplinary team providing the care. Such a review will immediately raise the key question of whose outcomes should have priority. Indeed, should there be reduced emphasis on clinical (perceptions of) outcomes and greater attention given to the user (perceptions of) outcome, even moving so far as allowing the patient's desired outcome to drive the disease management process? One can then move on to identify available measuring instruments and to select the most appropriate ones, bearing in mind evidence on reliability, validity and responsiveness to patient and clinically significant change, as well as acceptability, ease of use and clinical utility.

Current clinical practice must be appraised (through, for example, the audit process) and compared with the emerging synthesis of the current research evidence on what works, when and with whom, moving on to explore ways to modify existing practice where appropriate. If evidence on effectiveness is lacking, further research is indicated. Finally, data on desired and achieved outcomes (including patient expectations) must be collected, allowing

Table 3. A step-by-step guide

Step One:	Choose the service, condition, intervention or package of care for review
Step Two:	Clarify and identify the desired health (care) outcomes
Step Three:	Explore the potential causes of the condition and causal pathways into the health care system
Step Four:	Review available evidence on effectiveness
Step Five:	Select appropriate ways to measure the desired outcome
Step Six:	Monitor and audit the service provided

the monitoring and auditing of the services provided. Emphasis lies on 'doing it the best way' given available resources and the current state of knowledge—what can be expected 'on the average'. The underlying theme is to enhance the quality of health care provided to users.

Outcomes and rheumatoid arthritis

With a chronic disease such as rheumatoid arthritis (RA), no single desired outcome nor outcome measure is universally appropriate. Indeed, health benefit and outcome must be perceived in terms of (temporarily) arresting or slowing down the progression of the disease, rather than recovery. Furthermore, it becomes increasingly important to identify the desired outcomes, at various stages of the disease process, for the patient and carer—for example, the impact and burden of the disease on the patient's functioning and quality of life—as well as the desired outcomes for the practitioners providing care and treatment (Table 4).

Practitioners need to establish what it is they do that benefits

Table 4. Possible desired outcomes

Health Commissioning/Population Level
- To ensure cost-effective services
- To raise awareness about the condition
- To facilitate early access to specialist care
- To ensure provision of high quality care and treatment
- To enable seamless care across the interface of primary and secondary services

Practitioner
- To limit stress on affected joints (chiropody)
- To maintain mobility/function (physiotherapy)
- To identify most appropriate aids in order to maintain independence (occupational therapy)
- To slow down the progression of the disease (physician)
- To provide easy access to care and advice in the context of a flare

Patient
- To relieve pain
- To maintain (increase) mobility
- User specified/defined

Carer
- To assist the patient to remain an independent life
- To have adequate support to cope as a carer

---

patients in terms of the package as a whole and the several components of that package at the many stages of the disease, using such
data to argue for services with purchasers and to audit the services
provided. It is important to recognise that a focus on outcome
does not mean, and should not be interpreted as, a focus on a final
end-result. Especially with a chronic disease such as rheumatoid
arthritis with multiple treatment options, care points and practitioners providing care, each stage or process of care or intervention will have an outcome(s). Data need to be captured on each of
these both to monitor the service provided—achieved outcomes—and to evaluate the relative effectiveness of different treatment options. At the same time, it is critical that data collection
does not become a burden either to the patient or the health care
provider. Possible measures of outcome must therefore inform the
patient-clinician interaction, to identify what to do next and to provide a summary (outcome) of what has been achieved so far.

Evidence on effectiveness

The clinical course of RA has been divided into three forms of presentation (Scott and Huskisson 1992). Firstly, there is 'progressive'
chronic disease, with an invariable trend towards progression. Secondly, there is 'intermittent' disease, involving brief attacks, often
lasting for up to a year and intermissions for a variable lengths of
time. Thirdly, there is 'explosive' or 'malignant' disease which is
often fatal. In terms of causes, it is unclear whether lifestyle
(except weight through dietary practices) or socio-economic factors play a significant role-raising doubts over effectiveness of any
preventive approach—as opposed to constitutional and genetic
factors. Finally, onset of the disease is not confined, though more
common, among the elderly. Such a picture complicates decisions
on treatment options, on what drugs to use when, with whom and
for how long.

   Much research has focused on the efficacy of drug therapies.
First line drug treatments include analgesics and non-steroidal
anti-inflammatory drugs (NSAIDs). These aim to alleviate pain and
stiffness. Side-effects inevitably occur. As to which NSAIDs to use,
the evidence is unclear. Gotzsche (1993) reviewed the potential
sources of bias in studies exploring the effect of NSAIDs on joint
count in patients with rheumatoid arthritis. He showed that the
effect size was related to trial design (active or placebo control),
sample size, duration of treatment, drop-out rate, the existence of
a wash-in period, drug and dose. The guidelines of the British

Society for Rheumatology and the Research Unit of the Royal College of Physicians (Hopkins and Scott, 1992) conclude that there is no reason to prefer one NSAID to another, recommending clinicians to 'use the agents with which they have most experience', with analgesics being used as an adjunct.

There is considerable debate about whether slow-acting antirheumatic drugs—also known as second line or disease modifying drugs such as gold, penicillamine, sulphasalazine, methrotrexate and anti-malarials—should be given early on in the course of the disease (Wilske and Healey, 1989; Hess and Luggen, 1989). Low dose methotrexate is highly potent and has demonstrated efficacy and tolerability in a number of short- and longer-term clinical trials (Felson *et al*, 1992; Manganelli and Triose Rioda,1993). It appears not to have hepatotoxicity over the first 2 or 3 years, but questions over its long-term tolerance remain to be clarified (Schnabel and Gross, 1994). Alarcon *et al* (1992) conclude from their meta-analysis that despite its efficacy the possible role of methotrexate in slowing disease progression more than other second line drugs, as determined radiologically, is evident only when compared with azathioprine. Two recent studies (Tugwell *et al*, 1995 and Kirwan *et al*, 1995) have indicated the potential of combining slow-acting anti-rheumatic drugs (Tugwell *et al*, 1995) and changing the timing of treatment towards early active intervention (Kirwan *et al*, 1995), though further longer-term studies are still required.

The generalisability of such findings to routine practice has, however, been queried. Pincus (1993) argues that standard randomised controlled trials may not be able to detect the potential advantages of combining second line drugs because of their short timeframe, patient selection and study size. Rochon *et al* (1993) also demonstrated that older persons were generally omitted from drug trials of NSAIDs, while representing a high proportion of the population who are treated by them. More broadly, Felson (1993) pointed to the range of outcome measures used in trials, even on the one clinical issue of disease severity. There is a clear need to use the same outcome across trials in order to allow comparison of different therapies.

Finally, consensus based guidelines have been developed for RA (Hopkins and Scott, 1992). By definition, they may have a loose basis on a systematic overview of the literature on what works. In addition, guidelines have been developed by the British Society of Rheumatology (undated) and Arthritis Care (1992, 1994a, 1994b). The latter points, for example, to the need for early referral to a rheumatoligist, the value of effective team work to meet patient needs, good communication such that a patient with a 'flare' can get in touch, and patient education. These guidelines on audit and quality emphasise the need for a systematic review of evidence on effectiveness, in relation to the different presentations of RA, with a view to optimising the outcome for patients.

Conclusion

Assessing outcomes is a challenging task for both practitioners and purchasers. This is particularly so in RA with multiple stages, variable course and inexorable progressive deterioration. The task is to explore not only the question of 'does it work?', informed by good quality research evidence, but also the question, 'but does it work here?', that is, within this multidisciplinary clinical context and practice. Thus, does the achieved outcome match that expected from research?

A number of points must be emphasised (Table 5): in particular,

1. Identifying outcome criteria: whose outcomes are to be assessed? Is it the patient's and the health practitioners'? These must then be incorporated into the standard/goal setting stage of the audit cycle.
2. Establishing indicators of the specified outcomes, and appropriate data collection processes with a view to collect data on desired outcomes.
3. Ensuring that the achieved outcomes can be attributed to the intervention itself. It is important at least to clarify and specify what other factors could have also influenced the achieved outcome.
4. Deciding on an appropriate timescale over which to assess the achievement of the desired outcome.

The range of different interest groups—patient, carer, primary

Table 5. Six key questions in exploring outcome

- What is the basic process? Describe tasks and activities
- What factors might bring about the end-state/change?
- Whose perspective(s) on outcomes will be explored?
- How will these outcomes be measured?
- How will the data be collected and analysed?
- What timescale should be explored?

caregiver, specialist, other members of the clinical team, pur-
chaser/commissioner and policy-maker—must not be ignored nor
subsumed into a simple focus on one to the exclusion of the
others. A long term commitment to evaluation as part of the routine provision of services is required with the underlying aim of
both outcomes assessment and provision of better patient care in
clinical practice.

2 | Searching the literature

Alison Brettle
*Information Manager, UK Clearing House on Health Outcomes,
Nuffield Institute for Health, University of Leeds*

Introduction

Information related to measuring health status and outcomes for any condition or topic area can be found in a variety of sources: clinical journals, health management journals and journals relating to quality assurance, in addition to books and grey literature (that which is not readily available via conventional publishing channels). Locating relevant material can be problematic. This chapter discusses electronic databases and paper-based bibliographies, two useful sources for locating material on measuring health status and outcomes in relation to rheumatoid arthritis (particularly in relation to locating journal articles). Problems involved in carrying out literature searches on this topic are also highlighted.

Potential sources of health status and outcomes literature

Electronic databases

There are a number of widely available databases containing medical and health care information which are potentially useful sources of outcomes information. These databases are available on-line, on CD-ROM or via the organisation responsible for creating them. They cover general and broad areas such as those listed in Table 1. Others have a more specific focus, for example, relating to complementary therapies or cancer. There are, however, no specialised databases of this nature relating to rheumatology.

Paper-based bibliographies

Paper-based bibliographies are another method of locating relevant material. These can be published as documents in their own

Table 1. Databases containing medical and health care information

MEDLINE. This is the database produced by the US National Library of Medicine, and as such has an American bias. It covers an extensive range of literature relating to all aspects of biomedicine and indexes articles from approximately 3,400 journal titles.

EMBASE. This is a database produced by Elsevier Science and provides access to literature on pharmacology and biomedicine. It has a more European focus than MEDLINE, indexing articles from approximately 3,500 journal titles.

CINAHL. The Cumulative Index to Nursing and Allied Health Literature, as its name suggests, covers journal articles in the nursing and related fields, but again has an American slant.

HEALTHPLAN. This database covers literature relating to health planning and administration of health care, again with an American focus.

HELMIS. This database covers literature relating to health and social care management. It is produced by the Information Resource Centre at the Nuffield Institute for Health, University of Leeds and has a mainly UK focus.

right or frequently appear as part of a book. They are not always listed as a bibliography, but often form part of an extensive list of references. In relation to measuring health status and outcomes, some bibliographies covering the broad topic of outcomes have been published, with some having large sections relating to rheumatology (Table 2).

Searching Medline

To illustrate some of the issues involved in searching computerised databases, a literature search of Medline was carried out in the

Table 2. Bibliographies useful for locating outcomes material

Berzon *et al* (1995) Quality of life bibliography and indexes: 1993 update. *Quality of Life Research* vol 4, pp 53-73.

World Health Organisation. Division of Mental Health (1994) *Quality of life assessment: an annotated bibliography*. Geneva: World Health Organisation, Division of Mental Health.

Bowling A (1995) Measuring disease: a review of disease specific quality of life measurement scales. Buckingham: Open University Press.*

Scott D (ed)(1992) The course and outcome of rheumatoid arthritis. London: Baillière Tindall.*

* These bibliographies are part of books

area of health status and rheumatoid arthritis. Medline was selected due to its comprehensive coverage and accessibility.

When carrying out searches of computerised databases it is advisable to outline a search strategy beforehand and consider the phrases and words which should be included in the search. Searching Medline 'free-text' (that is, on relevant words or phrases which may appear anywhere in an article) can result in retrieving much irrelevant information since words such as 'outcome' are in common usage in many different contexts. An efficient method of retrieving manageable and relevant material is to use the Medline thesaurus: MeSH (Hall and Warburton, 1993). The thesaurus is a controlled list of terms applied to each article on the database to describe the concepts in each article. It provides a relatively easy means of retrieving all records discussing a subject of interest. Experience in searching Medline at the UK Clearing House has shown that the following terms identify relevant material when locating health status and outcomes documents.

health status

or

health status indicators

or

outcome and process assessment (health care)

or

quality of life

These terms can then be combined with the appropriate term for the subject area, in this case rheumatoid arthritis.

arthritis, rheumatoid (include all subject headings)

When a search of this nature has been carried out, a list of relevant documents should be retrieved. The information gained should look similar to that presented in Figure 1.

When carrying out a search on a database with a wide subject coverage such as Medline it is tempting to believe that the search has located all or most of the literature written on the subject of interest, particularly if the search strategy has been well thought out and has retrieved a high number of relevant articles.

Cross checking the search with another source can show that this is not the case. In this example, cross checking the Medline search with the material listed in a bibliography (Berzon *et al*, 1995) showed that the search failed to retrieve several important articles.

Two possible conclusions were drawn from this: the strategy was

```
UI   - 88120734
AU   - Affleck JW, Aitken RC, Hunter JA, McGuire RJ, Roy CW
IN   - Rehabilitation Studies Unit, Princess Margaret Rose Hospital,
       Edinburgh.
TI   - Rehabilitation status: a measure of medicosocial dysfunction.
SO   - Lancet 1988 Jan 30;1(8579):230-3
MH   - Activities of Daily Living, Adaptation, Psychological, Aged
MH   - Dependency (Psychology), Evaluation Studies, Factor Analysis,
       Statistical, Female, Health Status Indicators, Health Surveys
MH   - Human, Life Style, Male, Rehabilitation/px [Psychology]
MH   - Social Isolation
AB   - The Edinburgh Rehabilitation Status Scale (ERSS) measures four
       dimensions in which changes may occur in the course of a disabling
       illness or during rehabilitation: independence; activity; social
       integration; and effects of symptoms on lifestyle. It provides a
       profile of measures, the scores of which can be summated to
       indicate the overall level of performance of individuals or
       groups. Studies of its inter-observer reliability and of its
       application in various disability groups indicate that the ERSS
       reliably defines the characteristics of individual patients and of
       groups. The scale can be used conveniently by professional staff
       working independently or by a multiprofessional rehabilitation
       team to assess status and changes in patients. It can also be used
       for measurement of the effectiveness of services and for purposes
       of research, teaching, and administration.
PT   - Journal Article.
```

Fig 1. Example of a Medline article

inappropriate, but if this is the case what is the optimum search strategy? Or, articles on measuring outcomes and health status on Medline are indexed insufficiently. This was found to be the case with literature on randomised controlled trials listed on Medline (Lefebvre, 1994). Further research in this area needs to be carried out, but the exercise highlights the importance of using more than one source of information.

Using bibliographies and indexes

To illustrate the issues involved in searching a second source, searches of the *'Quality of life bibliographies and indexes'* (Berzon *et al*, 1995) were also carried out. They include papers or publications which have health-related quality of life measures as a significant focus. More explicitly papers were included if they:

- provided a theoretical explanation of the health related quality of life concept being applied,
- rationalised instrument selection within context of use,
- offered some evidence of psychometric properties.

Papers were identified utilising 'standard bibliographic searching techniques', (although these were not defined or the sources listed), from the authors' own reading and via readers' suggestions of additions to previous issues of the bibliography.

Bibliographies are more difficult and slower to use than computerised databases. They often have a more selective coverage, either by setting out inclusion criteria or in the case of reference lists in books highlighting those of particular interest or use to the author. In this case, papers are arranged alphabetically by first author. Within the bibliography papers can be found by making use of one of the indexes (instruments, therapeutic category and a cumulative index of instruments by therapeutic category).

Issues surrounding the choice and use of sources

The experience gained from the literature search on measuring health status and outcomes has shown that there are advantages and disadvantages in using both sources.

Computerised databases are relatively quick and easy to use and often provide an abstract of the article enabling the user to decide on its relevance without tracking down the article itself. Additionally, anyone can replicate or build on the search in the future to advance or update the work. On the other hand, not all relevant articles may be retrieved by the search strategy because of problems with the strategy itself or the way articles have been indexed for inclusion on the database.

In comparison, bibliographies can be more difficult to use. However, as they usually focus on one area all or many items may be relevant. There is no need to formulate a search strategy or worry about not retrieving items of interest. Nevertheless, the way the bibliography has been compiled and its inclusion criteria can ensure that some papers are not included in the bibliography at all. The structure of the indexes can make it difficult to locate papers.

Each approach has its own strengths and weaknesses; therefore it is essential not to rely on one method alone. If trying to carry out a comprehensive search and gain as much information about a subject as possible, it is necessary to use as many sources as are accessible. If possible, experts in the field should also be consulted to see if any important material has been missed. In addition, when carrying out the search of a computerised database more than one person should be involved; an information scientist or librarian—who will have the necessary information retrieval skills to carry out an effective search—and a clinical practitioner or researcher in the area of study—to gain expertise in the terminology and issues involved in the subject.

Future work

Although the two methods used retrieved over 173 records from 1980 onwards, this was the first step in carrying out a comprehensive literature search. The next stage is to carry out further searches using the other sources identified. Experts and practitioners working in the field need to be contacted, to identify other possible references and grey (unpublished or locally published) literature. As a further step, to make the retrieved records easily accessible, the material could be classified and published as a bibliography/document in its own right in hard copy and disk form (using a text retrieval database package or reference management software). Classification could be carried out in various ways, by author or subject or title, or by all three methods. Possible subject areas could build on the themes of this monograph; *domain* (functional, pain, psychological, quality of life, radiological, social) or *perspective* (clinician, economic, organisational, user-defined, trial, validation).

Conclusion

This chapter has aimed to highlight the range of sources which can be used in tracking down literature on measuring health status and outcomes, with particular reference to rheumatoid arthritis. A literature search carried out on this topic highlighted some of the issues involved in selecting sources of information. It is important not to confine the search to one source, rather use as many sources as are accessible. It is also important to draw on the experience of a number of people; information scientists, clinicians and/or researchers with expertise in the area of interest should be involved.

3 | A methodological perspective

Paul Dixon
Senior Research Fellow, UK Clearing House on Health Outcomes,
Nuffield Institute for Health, University of Leeds

Introduction

The outcomes of health care are measured with a wide range of methods and instruments. Measurements are needed for topics as varied as competency in self-medication and self-monitoring, all types of handicap, basic physical impairments, quality of life in many settings and much else besides. For any condition group or service, the ability of the available instruments to cover the range of possible outcomes is a crucial factor in the development of outcomes measurement. Rheumatoid arthritis (RA) care seems relatively fortunate in this respect. Not only are there instruments specifically developed to measure health status, but work is well advanced on charting the relation between these and established clinical measures such as erythrocyte sedimentation rate (ESR), radiographic scores and joint motion, swelling and tenderness (Pincus and Callaghan, 1992). Research is even beginning to tackle the difficult question of how the different measures might be used to explore the relation between patient and clinician views of significant change in the condition (Wells *et al*, 1993).

Later pieces in this collection give details of this work and the progress being made in specific forms of measurement for RA. This chapter has a broader focus. It highlights five widely recurring practical and methodological questions with particular relevance to measuring the quality of life and health status as RA outcomes, namely:

1. How can measurements reflect the needs of different settings and interests?
2. What emphasis should be placed on patient-defined outcomes and criteria for 'patient centredness'?
3. Should condition specific and/or multidimensional health status (generic) measures be used?

4. How should the basic methodological criteria be interpreted and applied in selecting instruments?
5. How appropriate are the methodological guidelines from clinical trials and other research to measuring the outcomes of routine care?

Measures and the settings for outcomes measurement

Many of the existing health status measures for outcomes work in rheumatoid arthritis have been tested and developed in clinical trials, for example, the Health Assessment Questionnaire (HAQ) and the Arthritis Impact Measurement Scale (AIMS). Though these measures have a relatively broad focus it is unclear how well they would meet the requirements of other settings or the interests of groups other than clinical researchers, for example, in how they would fare in:

- routine clinical practice;
- research to assess the effectiveness of different patterns of care delivery, including measuring the contribution of particular elements such as physiotherapy services;
- monitoring the quality of existing services;
- estimating the health gain provided by routine care (and related questions of particular interest to purchasers);
- recording and responding to patient-defined views of problems and outcomes.

The possibility of using what are predominately research-based instruments to measure the outcomes of routine care is probably the most pressing of these questions. At the risk of caricature, measurements developed for research can be very precise and capable of detecting small changes in health, but may be costly, time-consuming, intrusive and stress the clinical rather than the user perspective. This may make them unsuitable for regular use in routine care, where in contrast short, standardised and minimally disruptive measurements are required but which still may have to address a broad range of topics.

The pressure to collect information on routine care partly derives from the expansion of clinical audit, but also from the introduction of internal market within the NHS and, most particularly, the purchaser's interest in outcomes. This also raises the question of whether purchasers need new forms of information on outcomes. Some of their needs are not new—a shared interest with clinical researchers in identifying what are the most efficacious interventions under experimental conditions. But purchasers have several other outcomes agendas including wanting information on the effectiveness of routine care, as well as on the comparative performance of providers. Such information may take a number of forms:

- Levels of adherence to recommended protocols and interventions—these are assumed to be proxies for future outcomes.
- Information on health gain—whether targets are met for good outcomes.
- Information on avoidable health loss—whether complications are minimised.

These are not necessarily the same outcomes measurements that are required by clinicians or provider managers. At the same time, if outcomes specifications are to be included in contracts, then suitable information is most likely to be forthcoming if providers are convinced of its relevance and validity, and if it is cheap and easy to collect.

Whether instruments from clinical research can be modified for use in routine care or to reflect the interests of purchasers is an open question. More generally, the development of new settings for measurement and the broadening of the range of groups interested in health outcomes has created needs for new types of measure. The different interests and uses associated with different settings may thus differ in respect of their requirements for:

- the range of measurements and variables,
- the constructs and approaches underlying the measurements,
- the acceptable cost and volume of data, and
- the optimum form of analysis and presentation of results.

Measurements to reflect patient interests

Just as research-based measurements may not always meet the needs of purchasers and the majority of providers, so they may not be especially relevant to the interests of patients. At the policy level, there is now a strong commitment for outcomes measurement to reflect patient concerns, to give patients an opportunity to report their experiences in their own terms, and to accumulate accessible and intelligible information on possibilities for patient involvement in decisions on treatment options.

Patient involvement in outcomes measurement may take several forms. At the most passive, there are traditional methods for surveying levels of satisfaction with present services—and for collecting outcomes information for internal use by clinicians. More proactive models include disseminating outcomes information wide-ly, to allow communities to become involved in evidence-based pur-chasing decisions. More radical still are approaches that measure outcomes in relation to targets set by patients (or jointly with clini-cians) and those that provide outcomes information to enable indi-viduals to choose between treatment options or different providers.

Alongside the different approaches to patient involvement are different perspectives on what constitutes patient centred measure-ments. Instruments described as patient centred may vary widely in their capacity to reflect consumers' interests and concerns. At one extreme, there are verbatim records obtained from relatively unstructured conversations and interviews or from other methods of eliciting people's own views in their own words. At the other, there are short standard questionnaires completed by patients but devised around the constructs of clinicians and researchers.

Though RA is at the forefront of developing ways of recording patient preference and patient defined outcomes, there is still much work to be done. Further, these developments face several obstacles, not least that they may be thought to provide informa-tion that is too 'soft' and subjective for research purposes, but also too expensive for regular use in routine care.

The role of generic measures of health status

Because of the established condition specific measures in rheuma-tology, the issue of generic (multidimensional health status) mea-surements may be less important here than for some other special-ties. The questions are whether or not to subscribe to the use and development of generic health status instruments such as the NHP, EuroQol and SF-36, and whether the individual instruments and overall philosophy can usefully contribute to outcomes measure-ment in RA. Table 1 lists some generic health status measures that have been used within RA and some of the better known condition specific instruments.

The merits and limits of the generic approaches continue to be widely debated (Dixon *et al*, 1994). Four points are particularly rel-evant here. Firstly, generics may be most appropriate to applica-tions at an early stage in developing outcomes work, where there is still a need to trawl for the full range of possible effects. This is not the case in RA where there is probably sufficient agreement on what represents significant outcomes. Secondly, the potentially shorter generic instruments can be an attractive off-the peg option

Table 1. Commonly used condition-specific and generic measures in RA

Condition specific	Generic	Generic supplements
AIMS	MHIQ	TYPE forms:
AIMS 2	NHP	7.1
HAQ	MOS	7.2
ARA FC	Family	
FSI	LF-149	
Katz	LF-113	
Lee	SF-20	
MACTAR/PET	SF-36	
TQ	SIP/FLP	

when there are no brief condition specific instruments for use in routine care. However, they may be less relevant and less sensitive to change than condition specific instruments of similar length. Thirdly, generic instruments offer the possibility of making health status comparisons across condition groups and settings. Of particular attraction to purchasers is their purported ability to facilitate comparisons of different interventions for different conditions performed by different providers. Whether this is the case is a matter of considerable debate (Dixon *et al*, 1994). Finally, generic instruments are, by definition, grounded in what are presumed to be universal constructs of health. This raises basic questions of what is meant by, and how to test for, validity.

General criteria for selecting measures

Part of the UK Clearing House's remit is to promote a systematic and rigorous approach to assessing health status measurement including the standard criteria of validity, reliability and responsiveness. The principal criteria used in assessing instruments for outcomes work are listed in Table 2. They are well described in detail in several texts such as Wade (1992), Wilkin *et al* (1992) and Bowling (1995). Many of the criteria and associated tests are far from conclusive, though the ways the results are described can give the misleading impression that they are.

The widely quoted definition of *validity* can be misleading since it describes only one of three rather different approaches to the topic that can be found in the literature. The definition is most appropriate when the property to be measured can be directly

Table 2. Standard methodological criteria for assessing measures

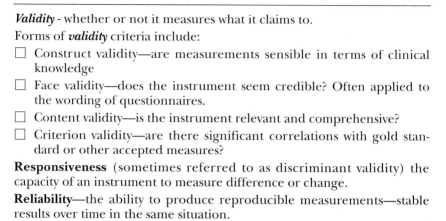

Validity - whether or not it measures what it claims to.

Forms of *validity* criteria include:

☐ Construct validity—are measurements sensible in terms of clinical knowledge

☐ Face validity—does the instrument seem credible? Often applied to the wording of questionnaires.

☐ Content validity—is the instrument relevant and comprehensive?

☐ Criterion validity—are there significant correlations with gold standard or other accepted measures?

Responsiveness (sometimes referred to as discriminant validity) the capacity of an instrument to measure difference or change.

Reliability—the ability to produce reproducible measurements—stable results over time in the same situation.

Other criteria—especially relevant to health status questionnaires, include *acceptability* and *intelligibility* to respondents.

---

defined. A second approach is harder to equate with the basic definition. This applies when there is no clear definition of what should be measured, but there is some idea of the factors with which the measurements should correlate, or factors that the measurements should predict. Measurements of social and physical functioning and self-report general health are three instances where this approach to validation is widely used. The relevant criterion is construct validity.

Even further from the basic definition are cases where validity testing relies on correlations with other instruments intended to measure similar things. The values of the correlations are frequently too low to do anything but refute the weak hypothesis that the instruments are unrelated; and this type of testing runs the risk of creating clusters of intercorrelated measurements of doubtful meaning. Criterion validity is the term used to describe this form of testing.

Responsiveness (the capacity to measure change or difference) is critical to outcomes measurement. The ability to measure change in an individual is the most demanding requirement for an instrument; it is far easier to detect large differences for the average health of large groups. Information on responsiveness is not widely available, nor information on what size difference is required or its meaning. The main dilemma is whether differences that are statistically significant are also clinically significant and would be perceived as significant by patients and carers.

The ability to produce reproducible measurements—stable results over time in the same situation—is described as *reliability*. The classic test, to take two measurements at the same time and place, is obviously impractical for many health status measurements, especially those based on questionnaires and other forms of self-report. An alternative test-retest procedure is used. This requires the measurement to be conducted on two occasions, separated by an interval that should be sufficiently long to minimise memory effects, but sufficiently short to reduce the likelihood of health having changed. This is also problematic and has led to an interest in approaches that examine features of the instrument that could cause unreliability. The best known are tests for internal consistency, that is, whether the items in an instrument (or its domains) are measuring the same thing.

However, internal consistency, often measured by Cronbach's alpha, is not the same as reliability. For certain types of instrument, high values of internal consistency should contribute to good reliability; though very high values probably mean that there is redundancy in the instrument, that is, several very similar questions. For instruments where scores summarise several different topics (multifactorial domains) the relation between internal consistency and reliability is uncertain, and high consistency could indicate invalidity. Once again, there is a need for caution when interpreting published data on reliability and internal consistency; a need not to get them confused; and a need to have a feel for the types of property that will be most relevant to the intended application.

Given the problems of applying the standard criteria, it is hardly surprising that there are many gaps in knowledge of the operating characteristics of most health status measures. More information is needed. But it is important to remember that statistical information on operating characteristics does not fully answer questions of what the measurements mean. It has been encouraging to note the prominence given in RA to discussions of face and content validity as well as to the more technical issues of criterion and construct validity. Hopefully future work will continue to maintain this balance between substantive and technical assessment.

Methods for measuring outcomes

Selecting a suitable measure is perhaps one of the easier aspects of outcome measurement. How to arrange the data collection so that there is a reasonable chance of inferring attribution is much more difficult. The procedures used to control confounders and facilitate attribution in randomised controlled trials and other experimental settings are well documented and well understood. The pressing issue is how far they can be adapted and adopted for use in routine care and, when they cannot, what other methods to use.

Evaluation research is grounded in the same methodology as experimental work, but it differs from research in more controlled settings in several ways. Firstly, there are limits to the design features that can be practically and ethically applied to routine care—double-blinding and withholding treatment from a control group are two of the more problematic. Secondly, evaluation research tends to address more operational and organisational questions. Thirdly, design issues are often resolved opportunistically: for example, when comparisons arise naturally where two similar groups of patients are receiving different treatments, or two providers organise similar services in different ways.

There is another approach which can be described as outcomes monitoring or outcomes audit. It aims to regularly collect outcomes information in routine settings, often as part of an audit dataset. It is difficult to generalise on the feasibility and most appropriate forms for this work. Measuring outcomes for chronic conditions is especially challenging. The key questions to resolve at the outset are what the intended outcomes for each phase of care are and what are the consequences for the timing and organisation of measurement. For example, is the aim to achieve stability over time, and if so, for how long? Is it to arrest decline, or even to achieve measuring short-term gain? Each implies different designs. Measuring change over time poses special problems, not least, as previously mentioned, the cost of instruments that are sufficiently sensitive. Key issues to resolve in each case include: what are key topics to measure as outcomes; what are appropriate markers of outcomes when it is not possible or practical to measure outcomes directly; what are the likely confounders; can these be measured and systematically accounted for; and what are appropriate points in time to make the measurements.

Conclusion

Research has a key role to play in informing all these issues and aiding the design of measurements for routine care. It would be a very considerable bonus if in addition to considering measurements for research purposes, attention could focus on providing some answers to some of the questions on how best to conduct routine outcomes measurement in RA.

4 | The rheumatologist's perspective

David V Doyle
Consultant Rheumatologist, Whipps Cross, Whipps Cross Road, London

Introduction

The rheumatologist has a different perspective for considering the outcome of rheumatoid arthritis (RA) from patients, purchasers, and other clinicians. A personal preference is to review the issues of assessing outcome in RA from three viewpoints: (a) problems relating to the rheumatoid disease process, (b) problems relating to the interpretation of treatment response; and (c) health status/quality of life measures. Each of these aspects will be considered in turn.

Problems relating to the disease process

What is RA? Epidemiological surveys suggest it is often a benign disease, which may enter prolonged remission or remit entirely. In a community based study of 4,522 individuals there were 118 who met the 1958 criteria for the classification of RA and had definite or probable disease. But at subsequent review 3–5 years later only 30 still had the disease. This meant that 73% no longer met the criteria for the diagnosis of RA (O'Sullivan and Cathcart, 1972).

In clinical practice there is a different picture, although this is not straightforward. In general RA appears as a persisting disease, which is severe and relentless in its progression. An example of outcome in early RA is seen in a report from Masi (1983) of a cohort study of 50 patients with RA seen within 6 months of the onset of symptoms. At baseline 38% were seropositive for rheumatoid factor. At 5 years 10% had no evidence of RA, 10% had severe progression and 80% had continuing disease.

Rheumatoid arthritis is characterised by progressive disability over time. Using the Stanford Health Assessment Questionnaire (HAQ) it has been clearly demonstrated that functional status

23

deteriorates over time. In a study of 1,274 patients it was found that disability occurred early in the course of the disease. Those patients with a disease duration of less than 6 months had a HAQ score approximately equal to that of the group as a whole whose mean duration of the disease was 7.4 years. At 12 years 50% had a HAQ score of greater than 1. At 6 years 50% had a HAQ score of greater than 2. At 10 years 50% had an HAQ score of greater than 2.5. Interestingly tender joint count, stiffness cause and ESR did not change over time despite this functional decline (Wolfe and Cathey, 1991; Wolfe *et al*, 1991).

Similar evidence of functional decline emerges from UK studies (Duthie *et al*, 1964; Scott *et al*, 1987). After 10 years of rheumatoid disease 30–40% of patients will fall into Steinbrocker functional class 3 or 4 (Steinbrocker *et al*, 1949). After 20 years 80% will be in these classes. The Bath study (Rasker and Cosh, 1984) suggested that after 11 years of rheumatoid arthritis 25% of individuals would be in Steinbrocker class 3 or 4 and after 15 years 50% would be in these groups.

There are several indicators of outcome. Older patients with rheumatoid tend to have a poorer outcome (Scott *et al*, 1987; Sherrer *et al*, 1987). Comorbidity is also likely to influence outcome adversely. Leigh and Fries (1992) looked at predictors of mortality in a rheumatoid community population over an 8 year period and have highlighted the following predictors: older age, male sex, single status, unemployed, poor education level, high HAQ score and steroid usage.

Several major patterns of disease have been documented (Short and Bauer, 1948; Short, 1968). In assessing what happens to an individual during a course of rheumatoid arthritis we may use health status measures. These should be able to reflect the impact produced by fluctuations in disease activity. We also need to be able to measure the ultimate outcome of the disease process. Even if we are to assume that the majority of patients have a similar end outcome there will be considerable variation in individual health status during the course of that disease process: some individuals flaring intermittently, others progressively deteriorating.

Problems in assessing treatment

Slow-acting anti-rheumatic drugs (SAARD) improve clinical and laboratory measures of rheumatoid arthritis in the short-term but there is doubt about their long-term effectiveness (Situnayake, 1988; Gabriel and Luthra, 1988). Lack of evidence of long-term benefit may be the result of high rates of treatment withdrawal over time (Wolfe *et al*, 1990). Using the ARAMIS database Singh *et al* (1991) found high rates of drug discontinuation in the first 6 months of starting a slow-acting anti-rheumatic drug. These varied from 15% for patients starting methotrexate and 17% for hydroxy-chloroquine to 48% of patients starting cyclophosphamide. The reasons why there is uncertainty about the long-term treatment response in RA are summarised in Table 1.

Table 1. Possible reasons for lack of long-term treatment response

---

1. Clinical trial patients are not representative of the rheumatoid population as a whole
2. Most studies last less than 12 months
3. In practice 50% of non-steroidal anti-inflammatory drugs and slow-
   acting anti-rheumatic drugs are discontinued within 1–2 years of
   initiation and 80% within 5 years

The traditional clinical and laboratory measures of treatment effectiveness that we use may be less than ideal. Long-term out-come studies show little change in ESR and rheumatoid factor titres over time despite functional deterioration. Slow-acting drugs improve traditional clinical measures of disease activity but have not been shown to halt functional decline. There is some evidence that functional disability in early rheumatoid arthritis is a consequence of inflammation, overall functional disability increases slowly and steadily and is less influenced by acute flare (Guillemin *et al*, 1992). Sex may also have an influence on functional ability. Thompson and Pegley (1991) have suggested that HAQ score is lower in women than in men for any given level of disease activity.

Remission is the ultimate aim of treatment. Wolfe and Hawley (1985) reported their experience in 485 patients given gold or penicillamine. After 6 months 18% were classified as achieving remission. But over the next 3 years less than 10% of these remissions were sustained. This meant that under 2% of those treated achieved a persistent remission.

Health status and quality of life issues

These assessment measures attempt to combine physical functioning and emotional functioning. In general they are as reliable and sensitive as traditional measures of improvement in clinical status (Mitchell *et al*, 1986). But there are several limitations of using quality of life measures to assess RA. First, a generic measure such as the SF-36 has few items relevant to upper limb function. Second, disease specific yardsticks such as the Arthritis Impact Measurement Scale (AIMS) do not allow inter-disease outcome comparisons to be made. Third, measurements of specific functions by questionnaire may be too crude for monitoring individual subjects (as opposed to epidemiological studies using groups of patients). Floor and ceiling effects inherent in many questionnaires mean that they are less accurate in portraying the patient at the top or bottom ends of the disability spectrum. Finally generally they may be difficult to use with children, the elderly and those with mental impairment or poor English.

More generally values change with time, people learn and adjust or accommodate to disability over the course of a long illness. These changes may alter the health status score even if objective function has not changed at all. Similarly health status values will be influenced by changes in personal circumstances, both social and economic. These alterations in health status score over time may hamper the longitudinal use of scales when used to assess, for example, the effectiveness of a particular drug treatment or treatment strategy.

An example of the effect of personal circumstances on outcome is shown in a small survey undertaken at Whipps Cross Hospital (Whipps Cross Survey. Johansen and Doyle, 1993). This compared an elderly and a younger population with rheumatoid disease of similar severity and duration. The older patient group had lower expectations of outcome when measured on the physical and mental health scales of SF-20 and tended to view themselves as less disabled by their rheumatoid disease than younger patients with similar physical disability (Table 2).

Table 2. Effect of age on satisfaction with rheumatoid outcome: results from the Whipps Cross Survey. (Johansen and Doyle, 1993)

	Aged under 65 years	Aged over 65 years	Difference
Mean age	55	73	
Number of patients	27	26	
Mean disease duration in years	12.1	10.9	
Mean HAQ	1.66	1.86	Not significant
Mean SF-20 subjective physical well-being	30.7	44.3	$p < 0.05$
Mean SF-20 mental well-being	59.9	68.8	$p < 0.05$

Conclusion

Outcome assessment for rheumatoid arthritis should include a range of measures: anthropometric measures; measures of physical function; and measures of health status. A framework for considering what yardsticks to use is shown in Table 3. These must reflect

Table 3. Framework for clinical outcome measures

Clinical state	Measurement
Disease assessment	Joint count, haemoglobin, ESR, C-reactive protein, rheumatoid factor
Impairment	Joint deformity, X-ray erosion
Disability	HAQ, functional class
Disability—handicap	Health status measures
Handicap	Work disability, time lost
Death	Mortality

the fact that variations in outcome of chronic diseases like rheumatoid are complex and are the result of many influences. Some of these influences are the consequence of disease severity but others are the result of social and environmental factors over which the rheumatologist has virtually no influence, for example, social, economic and educational status. Rheumatologists and health planners need to take into consideration these particular problems when interpreting data obtained on rheumatoid arthritis.

A number of developments of health status measures are needed. First, it may be important to develop specific items to assess disability for individual rheumatic disease. For example, upper limb function needs assessment in the rheumatoid patient, spinal function in the patient with ankylosing spondylitis. Second, there should be greater priority given to the views of patients about their disease outcomes. This includes improved assessment of patient satisfaction with health status and treatment. Finally, it is important to identify specific thresholds of health status at which intervention might make a difference, for example, the point at which hip replacement would be advantageous or the point at which initiation of a new slow-acting drug might be effective.

5 | A patient's perspective

Jean Ashcroft
Director of Policy and Campaigning, Arthritis Care, London

Background

Unlike many chronic long-term medical conditions most people, irrespective of their age, will have heard the term 'arthritis'. Many of those people will also know of at least one person with arthritis. That person may even be a close family member, friend or neighbour.

For me, it was an elderly neighbour with rheumatoid arthritis (RA) and like most people prior to the onset of my own RA, I would frequently discuss her situation with my own family, neighbours, work colleagues, and anyone else, should the opportunity arise. I was, of course like most people, very judgmental in what I said—'she really doesn't try hard enough, she just sits there all day doing nothing but watch the television. She made her sister get up early every morning and visit her—in all winds and weather, so that she can have her breakfast in bed, prepare her meals for the rest of the day, and do her housework—but she can go off to bingo all right in the evening!'

I did my neighbourly bit, and often stood in at weekends to give her sister a break. My husband and I responded to the all too frequent cries for help, and of course felt good about it! When she finally died, I declared it was a happy release, as 'she didn't have much of a life anyway, and was after all a total burden on her sister!'

Little was I to know that two years on I would wake up one morning and find I had extreme difficulty getting out of bed due to pain and stiffness in both knees and also in the joints of both hands, which made routine early morning tasks, like squeezing the toothpaste and lifting the kettle very painful and difficult.

Having finally struggled to wash and dress I would force myself into continuing with the daily routine of going to work. Once there, I began to experience great difficulty in going up and down the stairs, writing, typing, filing and generally keeping pace with my work colleagues, everything was so painful, and I was so slow. The full impact of the initial stage of the disease process is, therefore, present long before the diagnosis has even been made, its disruptive nature is already beginning to control what you can and can't do.

Negative images of RA—negative outcomes

Is it no wonder then that diagnosis itself is so often welcomed, not only by the individual, but also their immediate family and friends. However, this initial welcoming is short lived as the reality begins to set in, bringing with it that nightmare of a mental picture that seems to overwhelm and haunt you. For me, it was of a little old lady, exactly like my neighbour, all crippled up, sitting all day in a wheelchair, unable to do anything, a total burden on her family, friends and neighbours—to say nothing of the State!

Sadly after 25 years, those negative images of people with RA still remain, and continue to haunt not only every newly diagnosed person, but also their family and friends. Sadder still, for many it even becomes reality!

Early diagnosis brings with it a never ending stream of appointments with consultants, doctors, occupational therapists, physiotherapists, blood tests, X-rays, trips to your GP and chemist, etc. This coupled with the extreme fatigue that accompanies RA leads to your entire life being absorbed within the medical world. It will undoubtedly begin with taking time off work, the odd morning here, afternoon there, be late in, leave early; your work will undoubtedly suffer, work colleagues will have to cover for you. To your employer and the outside world you are, unwittingly, contributing to that negative image of disability. Even worse still you begin to see yourself as being a burden, your sense of worth is being destroyed, and with it will go your self-esteem.

Family life becomes affected—can't make the children's sports day, can't collect them from school on Wednesday or Friday this week, can't make that lunch date with a friend, have to cancel the long weekend break away because you have a hospital appointment at 9 o'clock on Monday morning. Children, family and friends see you, 'as always being ill', 'unreliable', 'can't plan anything'. They stop asking you to join them in their activities, you become depressed and as a consequence your family becomes depressed.

All of the above represents the insidious nature of RA at its very best, sucking you very quickly into an 'illness mode'—the 'medical model of disability', and like most things held in by suction, it is very difficult, if not impossible to get back out.

Health professional defined outcomes

Health professionals measure the health status of people with RA in a variety of different ways, aimed initially at establishing 'what works on whom, and why'. Some accept that there is a need to consider and take into account the impact of the disease on the individual's social functioning (Long and Scott, 1994). Few, if any, carry this forward, due in the main to their tradition of working entirely within the medical model of disability.

The medical model of disability is the birthplace of the negative images that surround disability. RA is no exception. It is, therefore, essential to recognise this within that very first appointment.

The results of this monitoring of patient's health status is increasingly being used to meet the needs of the NHS purchaser–provider environment, thus resulting in the perpetuation of the medical model of disability and all the negativity that surrounds it.

Patient defined outcomes

RA is a long-term medical condition. It will make its presence known each and every day for the rest of your life. The overall impact of that presence will largely be determined by the patient's understanding of the illness process, the sharing of that understanding with immediate family and friends, and the way in which not only your treatment, but also the monitoring of that treatment, is being delivered to you.

A major contributor to successful outcomes in RA is, without doubt, patient education programmes. Arthritis Care is actively involved in the delivery of such programmes within its 'Self-Help Initiatives Project' (SHIP) (Jones and Crutchley). This includes the Arthritis Self Management Programme (ASMP) (Lorig and Fries, 1995). Through these programmes a 'new generation' of patient is rapidly emerging, patients who have been totally empowered following courses on self-help, self-management and personal development, resulting in renewed self-esteem and a sense of real worth which in turn is enabling patients for the first time in many years to take control, not only of their lives, but also of their disease.

Once that control has been achieved and maintained you will have the key to successful, 'patient defined' outcomes. It is, therefore, essential from day one of diagnosis that all health professionals involved in the delivery of education and treatment recognise the potential of such courses.

Patient-led services and delivery

Arthritis Care, in consultation with the British League Against Rheumatism, has produced a set of *Quality Guidelines* on primary health care (Arthritis Care, 1992), secondary health care (Arthritis Care, 1994a) and community health care (Arthritis Care, 1994b). These guidelines also form part of the British League Against Rheumatism (1994) 'Purchasers Pack'. All need to be adopted by purchasers and to inform the delivery of health care.

If the full consequences of the disabling and destructive impact of arthritis, not only on the individual concerned, but also on their immediate family and friends is to be avoided, it is essential that all health professionals see their patients as 'equal partners' (Smith, 1995) and include them in the decision-making process on the choice of treatments available, including the timing of surgical procedures, which in turn will greatly enhance overall outcome.

Service delivery should be timely, taking into account the domestic, social, work/education and leisure needs of each individual person. To achieve this all health professionals responsible for the purchasing and delivery of such services should undertake to establish the 'social needs' of each individual person. Once established this should be reviewed on an annual basis, unless individual circumstances determine otherwise. It should form part of the overall monitoring procedures which are already in place in many rheumatology clinics.

Particular attention should be given to maintaining the individual person in their existing educational or working environment. A change in the attitude of doctors is therefore essential:

- Rather than condoning a slide into disability and dependency, they should see maintaining the person in education or employment as their priority (Ellis, 1995).
- Routine appointments, particularly for monitoring side-effects of drugs and the disease process, must, therefore, be in full consultation with the person concerned. This may mean providing evening and weekend clinics for blood tests, injections, infusions, etc.
- Joint replacement surgery and other non-urgent 'in hospital'

treatments must be carried out when it best suits the individual person.

- All rheumatology services should have an information system which provides information on waiting times for routine non-urgent appointments (Smith, 1995), thus enabling the individual to negotiate the most convenient time for surgery to take place.

In addition to the above, existing working arrangements in rheumatology departments should be organised to ensure people with arthritis receive health care appropriate to their needs. This means reviewing the roles of rheumatologists, rheumatology nurse practitioners and all other health professionals involved to ensure the most effective use is being made of each relative to the needs of the patient. Arthritis Care is aware that different approaches are being pursued in different hospitals and would urge that steps be taken to assess their relative effectiveness (British Society for Rheumatology).

Occupational therapy assessments should take place in the home, at a time convenient to the family concerned. It should not, however, restrict itself to identifying and meeting those needs that occur only in the home. All aspects of need must be taken fully into account. This may well lead to working with other colleagues within the Departments of Employment or Education.

Most broadly, health commissioning agencies, together with GPs, should encourage and support joint initiatives by health providers and social service departments to ensure that the concept of a seamless service can be realised in practice (Arthritis Care, 1994b).

Conclusion

Am I a patient or a person? The answer is quite simple. I am a patient only when I am in hospital, attending a rheumatology or orthopaedic outpatients clinic, a physiotherapy session, my GP etc. If, however, I am to remain in control of my RA it is essential that no more than 25% of my time is taken up as a patient. For every 1% of my time above that limit I start to lose control of my life, when it reaches 51% it has gained a majority share and has effectively succeeded in its bid to take over my life entirely. Once that has happened health professionals, not me or my family, friends and work colleagues, are the majority shareholders in my life.

Having RA is very time consuming, not least because by its very nature you carry out everyday tasks at a slower pace than your non-disabled colleagues. It is, therefore, essential that in addition to ensuring that I only spend 25% of my time attending to its ever increasing medical demands, that I do so within a framework that promotes positive outcomes, reduces dependency, and does not see disability as a negative experience. Promoting the positive acceptance and use of disability equipment within the social model of disability both empowers and enables disabled people, thus enabling us to take our rightful place as equal citizens in our society. That is the 'one and only outcome' that we should all be seeking to achieve.

6 | An overview of studies of disease outcome

David L Scott
Reader in Rheumatology, Department of Rheumatology, King's College Hospital, London

and

Andrew F Long
Project Leader, UK Clearing House on Health Outcomes, Nuffield Institute for Health, University of Leeds

Introduction

A paradox at the centre of the treatment of rheumatoid arthritis (RA) was delineated by Pincus (1992). Short-term studies of anti-rheumatic therapy invariably show it is successful while long-term outcome of the disease is poor. Several factors underlie this paradox. Results of therapies for RA are usually evaluated in clinical trials over short periods rather than as long-term clinical observations over many years. Increased mortality rates often go unrecognised. Further, reports indicating an optimistic prognosis are often based on epidemiological studies rather than patients in clinical settings. In such studies there are many patients with mild RA who have no evidence of disease 3 to 5 years later. By contrast, in clinical settings more than 90% of patients with RA have evidence of disease 3 to 5 years later, generally with progression.

It is against this paradox that this review is situated. It aims to provide a summary of available literature on outcome for patients with RA. In so doing, it attempts to explain Pincus' paradox and to introduce some of the complexities surrounding the issue of monitoring and assessing disease outcome in RA.

Evidence on outcome for different patient groups

The many outcome studies in the area have not evaluated similar patient groups. Some studies have focused on hospital patient populations—either as in- or outpatient settings—regional studies and population surveys.

There are four major morbidity studies of patients with RA initially seen as hospital inpatients (Short *et al,* 1957; Duthie *et al,* 1964; Amor *et al,* 1981; Scott *et al,* 1987) including between 100 and 307 cases, all selected because they needed hospital admission. The Boston series (Short *et al,* 1957) looked at patients first seen between 1931 and 1936, while the Droitwich series (Scott *et al,* 1987) studied patients initially seen from 1966 to 1968. Steinbrocker functional classes (Steinbrocker, Traeger and Batterman, 1949) were used in both studies. After 10 years, the Droitwich and Edinburgh series (Scott *et al,* 1987; Duthie *et al,* 1964) reported that 30–40% of patients were in Steinbrocker functional classes 3 or 4 (off work or housebound); after 20 years, 80% of patients were in these classes.

Hospital outpatient studies have been reported from New York (Ragan and Farringdom, 1962), Bath (Rasker and Cosh, 1984) and Nashville (Pincus *et al,* 1984). The Bath series describes 20-year results for 100 consecutive rheumatoid patients seen within one year of presentation. At 15 years, of the 65 patients who were still alive, 51% were in Steinbrocker functional class 3 or 4. At 20 years, of the 54 patients who were still alive, 45% were in classes 3 and 4. Similar results were seen in New York, with 50% of 246 patients being in these classes after 13 years of observation.

In contrast to these hospital patient studies, a regional survey from Saskatchewan (Sherrer *et al,* 1986) found that after nearly 12 years 36% of the 681 patients were in functional classes 3 or 4. Disability, measured by the Health Assessment Questionnaire (HAQ), developed most rapidly during the first years after disease onset and assumed a slow, nearly linear rate of increase after 10 years. The worst prognosis was seen in older women who showed radiological worsening and developed functional impairment early in the disease. Approximately 10% of the patients developed significant disability.

Finally, a recent study reviewed 64 survivors from a prospective study of early rheumatoid disease (Corbett *et al,* 1993) at a mean of 15 years from presentation. They were compared with 29 patients who had died. There was a small increase in mortality due to the disease itself, but only one death was directly caused by it. One-fifth at entry to the study, and two-fifths by the time of death, had poor functional capacity. Of 64 survivors, six had poor functional capacity at entry and nine after 15 years. Almost 60% of survivors remained with or improved to normal function at 15 years. This study suggested morbidity is not as bad as has been generally considered.

It is evident that the patient group studied has a considerable influence on the observed outcome. Cases selected from the general population invariably do best. In general, 80% of cases first seen as hospital inpatients will be moderately or severely impaired and disabled after 20 years in contrast to about 20% of patients selected from the general population. The average outpatient with RA has a 30% chance of becoming severely disabled.

Assessment of disease activity

Understanding the approaches in the assessment of disease activity in RA is important to understanding its outcome. It has been an area of intense contemporary investigation. Determining joint involvement is especially important. Prevoo *et al* (1993) contrasted several available methods, including the Ritchie index (Ritchie *et al*, 1968), a modified Ritchie index, the Thompson-Kirwan index (Thompson *et al*, 1987), the 28 joint index, the 36 joint index, total tender joints, and total swollen joints. They found that the seven indices studied had similar reliability and validity; no joint index was thus superior for measuring disease activity. Fuchs and Pincus (1994) also showed assessment of a reduced number of joints provides information equivalent to that obtained by the traditional 60-joint evaluation. The effect sizes of the joint scores derived using a reduced number of joints were similar to those of the original 60-joint score.

European collaboration across multiple centres (Scott *et al*, 1992; 1993) has concluded that the best measures to assess RA are: the number of swollen joints, the number of tender joints, and the ESR. This supports work of van der Heijde *et al* (1990) who showed the best single variable to be the number of swollen joints and the best composite index the disease activity score. This latter score was derived from the number of swollen joints, the number of tender joints and the ESR. Fuchs (1993) found that the disease activity score provides a simple and effective measure of inflammation and discriminates drug from placebo treated patients.

The ideal minimum data set has also been defined (Felson *et al*, 1993). It consists of the number of tender joints, the number of swollen joints, articular pain, ESR, and patients' and physicians' (assessors') global judgement of disease activity. There should also be an assessment of function; a simplified measure needed which can then be translated into all European languages.

Factors predicting outcome

A wide range of factors have been uncovered within research studies on RA patients as predicting the outcome of the disease. Age, gender and disease duration predict outcome (Sherrer *et al*, 1987). This study of 2,448 patients seen at three North American centres also found that the initial level of disability and radiographic assessments of joint damage were also good predictors of subsequent disability, while elevated ESRs and rheumatoid factor titres—though associated with future disability—had a non-linear relationship and were less useful in predicting disease outcome. Kaarela's (1985) study of 442 patients with recent arthritis compared 22 variables recorded at the onset of arthritis in patients with RA and related these to the subsequent outcome of the disease. Outcome data was collected on only 200 of the cases. Of these, half had a poor outcome. He concluded that a destructive form of arthritis is best indicated at the onset of an inflammatory synovitis by the presence of: a symmetrical polyarthritis of peripheral joints, serum rheumatoid factor, morning stiffness, high ESR, and old age.

Rheumatoid factor is an important indicator of progression. Isomaki (1987) reviewed follow-up results of unselected adult arthritis cases. The outcome was worst at 8 years in seropositive rheumatoid patients and best in seronegative oligoarthritis of unknown aetiology. The outcome of seronegative arthritis was bimodal: a majority of cases had a favourable outcome but a minority did not do well. Reilly *et al* (1988) compared the need for therapy in seropositive and seronegative cases. Seronegative males were less likely to require slow-acting drugs than seropositive males: there were no differences in the requirements for slow-acting drugs in seropositive and seronegative females. Seronegative disease had a broadly similar outcome to seropositive RA in this referral-centre population.

Measures of functional disability such as the button test, modified walking time, and responses to a questionnaire about activities of daily living have been related to outcome (Pincus *et al*, 1987) and are all weak predictors. Formal educational level is also related to morbidity. Callahan and Pincus (1988) have shown that clinical status measures such as the ESR and joint count are worse in patients who did not complete high school.

Although RA is related to HLA DR4 there is little evidence it is a useful predictor of outcome. Silman *et al* (1986) followed 59 rheumatoid patients first seen with early disease and followed them for 3 years. They found no evidence that HLA DR4 was a useful indicator of subsequent outcome. There is also no evidence that HLA antigens predict response to anti-rheumatic drug therapy. Moens *et al* (1987) showed HLA typing was not useful in predicting

the outcome of treatment with penicillamine in a study of 111 consecutive cases treated with this drug and followed for 7–9 years.
Further evidence that single measures of disease activity do not
predict outcome is provided by Hassell *et al* (1993) who evaluated
disease activity measured annually over 7 years in 127 patients.
They studied the relationship of serial measures of disease activity
(looking at the area under the curve for each variable followed
with time) to outcome measured radiologically, functionally and by
global assessment. A significant correlation was found between
persistent disease activity and radiographic deterioration. Similar
results were found for functional outcome measured by Steinbrocker grade, health assessment questionnaire score or global
assessment (by analogue score).

Overall patients with the most severe RA have the worst prognosis. This group includes those with a persistently high ESR, strongly
positive tests for rheumatoid factor, and severe extra-articular disease. Age and gender influence outcome, with older women having a less favourable outcome. Notwithstanding, there is a subgroup of elderly patients who have a more favourable outlook.
They often have a polymyalgic onset of their arthritis and may have
a disease variant. For example, Deal *et al* (1985), in a study of 78
patients presenting with RA after the age of 60 years compared to
134 cases whose disease onset was at a younger age, found that
only 48% of the elderly patients were seropositive for rheumatoid
factor compared to 76% of the younger age group.

Recent studies on prognostic markers

Research into prognostic factors has explored the role of several
potential predictors of outcome. Age and rheumatoid factor status
are important (van-Schaardenburg *et al*, 1993). Van Zeben *et al*
(1993) in their study of prognostic factors in 132 RA patients followed from an early phase of the disease (symptoms <5 years) for 6
years, used a combination of three commonly available variables
(number of swollen joints, IgM-rheumatoid factor and the erosion
score). They showed that these closely approximated the maximal
accuracy that could be achieved with a larger number of variables.
This confirmed their earlier study which found increased rheumatoid factor levels in early RA, especially a high level of IgA RF within 3 years of the onset of symptoms, was prognostic for a more
severe disease outcome 6 years after the onset of symptoms (Van
Zeben *et al*, 1992).

Demographic, clinical, laboratory and genetic features and

radiographic damage at onset has also been found to affect the outcome after 2 years. Van der Heijde *et al,* (1992), in a prospective study of 147 patients, showed that radiographic damage after 2 years was predicted by high disease activity at the start (measured as erythrocyte sedimentation rate, C-reactive protein or Disease Activity Score) combined with DR4 or DR2 (as a prognostically favourable factor) and rheumatoid factor positivity. Radiographic damage was better predicted if disease activity during the first 6 months was included. Absence or presence of progression of radiographic damage could be correctly predicted in 83% of the patients.

Patient scores on the Health Assessment Questionnaire have predictive value. Leigh and Fries (1992) used the HAQ to identify predictors of outcome in an 8 year study of 330 patients. The initial level of this disability index was by far the strongest predictive variable and provided a clinically important gauge for the likelihood of future impairment.

The prognostic value of an impaired ability to oxidise sulphur was examined by Emery *et al* (1992) in 54 patients with recent onset symmetrical polyarthritis who were followed up at 1 and 4 years. Those patients with persistent disease at 1 year had a prevalence of poor S-oxidation of 69%. At 4 years 74% of those with a diagnosis of RA were poor S-oxidisers compared to 31% of those who were asymptomatic. A defective ability to oxidise sulphur appears to predispose to persistent clinical disease. Another study of early RA by Paimela *et al* (1993) followed 87 patients with early RA for 3 years. Following anti-rheumatic treatment, a similar improvement in clinical variables and laboratory measure assessing disease activity was found in both DR4-positive and DR4-negative RA patients. This suggests DR-4 status is of limited relevance in prognosis of early RA.

Recent studies of anti-rheumatic drugs and outcome

Pincus (1993) highlighted the limitations of randomised controlled clinical trials. Their drawbacks include: excessive attention to group data rather than individual patient responses; many exclusion criteria which ignore a large part of the RA population; small study numbers with insufficient statistical power to identify clinically important trends; and a timeframe too short to recognise clinically meaningful differences between treatment regimens. The long-term outcome of sequential monotherapy based on the therapeutic pyramid has been disappointing. A review of prognostic factors, acute disease activity measures, functional measures, and the results of preliminary trials with combination therapy by Wilke *et al* (1993) suggest specific goals of treatment can be established and that logical, aggressive treatment in early disease can be accomplished. These goals should include prompt control and continuous reduction of the active joint count.

The comparative merits of commonly used disease-modifying drugs in the treatment of RA and the influence of age, gender, and disease duration on the outcome of treatment was assessed by Capell *et al* (1993). Gold, penicillamine and sulphasalazine performed similarly, with about 60% of patients continuing to receive each of these drugs for at least one year. Neither gender nor age influenced the response to treatment, but patients with a longer disease duration showed a greater tendency to stop treatment. The median percentage improvement was 33% in pain score and 50% in ESR.

There have been several studies of methotrexate. Kremer and Phelps (1992) reported its use in a cohort of RA patients receiving weekly oral methotrexate for 90 months. A significant improvement from baseline was maintained in all clinical parameters except the number of tender joints. Toxic reactions were equally common early and late in treatment. Radiographic scores for erosive disease became statistically significantly different from baseline at year 8. Weinblatt *et al* (1992) determined the long-term efficacy and safety of low-dose methotrexate in RA in an 84 month open prospective study of 26 cases. A significant improvement was demonstrated after 36 months therapy. Twelve patients were treated for 84 months. They maintained improvements in painful joints, swollen joints, pain, and physician and patient global assessments. At 84 months, 46% of the patients remained in the study. Tishler *et al* (1993) described changes in 126 RA patients treated with low doses of methotrexate for 3 years or more. The overall probability of continuing with therapy was 72% at 2 and 3 years and 65% at 5–7 years. Out of the whole group 45% experienced marked improvement and 6% achieved clinical remission. Alarcon *et al* (1992) reviewed the clinical and radiological effects of methotrexate. They felt it is efficacious but its effects on X-ray progression are open to question. They performed a meta-analysis of 353 methotrexate treated and 205 controls and computed a monthly rate of disease progression. The rates of disease progression were similar for methotrexate treated cases and controls.

Cyclosporin can now be used to treat RA. Wells and Tugwell (1993) reviewed its use in five prospective clinical trials. A composite effect score for efficacy and the rates of dropout due to toxicity were each compared to earlier meta-analyses evaluating the relative efficacy and toxicity of second-line drugs for RA. The composite effect for cyclosporin indicated significant improvement over placebo. This effect in excess of placebo was in the range of that found for antimalarial drugs and its associated toxicity was similar to that found with drugs with low toxicity, such as auranofin.

Several studies have looked at the effects of gold injections. Epstein *et al* (1991) evaluated the results of gold on the course of RA over a 5 year period in 822 patients seen in a community setting. The two main outcome variables were the Health Assessment Questionnaire and the number of painful joints. There was no convincing evidence for change in the course of RA over the 5 years. This rather negative view of the effects of gold was contradicted by a longer study from Lehtinen and Isomaki (1991) of 573 RA patients first treated between 1961 and 1966; 520 were given gold for varying durations. By 1989 251 patients had died. The mortality was least in those who had been given gold for at least 10 years and survival was least in those who had never had gold. Wolfe *et al* (1993) also provided a more positive perspective of the efficacy of gold in clinical practice. Ninety-eight RA patients treated for at least 1 year were studied. Assessments included joint counts, erythrocyte sedimentation rate, and morning stiffness. All outcome measures showed significant improvements at one year. Important improvement was common: joint counts fell by 63%, ESR by 48%, and morning stiffness by 72%. Overall improvement was equivalent of 2 months without pain or disability.

Finally, there has been recent interest in both early treatment and combination therapy with two slow-acting drugs. Kirwan et al (1995) have shown that the early use of oral steroids combined with a slow-acting drug in active disease slows down the progression of joint damage assessed radiologically. Tugwell *et al* (1995) showed that combining methotrexate and cyclosporin was more effective in controlling the disease than therapy with a single agent. These studies suggest that new therapeutic approaches with conventional drugs may be beneficial. It is an important area for further investigation.

Conclusion

Specialist rheumatology practice is changing. Large inpatient units in spa hospitals have closed, for example Highfield Hospital at Droitwich. Clinical services are outpatient focused and linked to

local primary care. There is increasing pressure for all new specialist referrals to be seen rapidly and the place of long-term specialist
care is increasingly questioned. The provision of specialist rheumatology services should be related to: the frequency of rheumatic
diseases in the population; the overall burden caused by these diseases; and the ability of patients to benefit from specialist health
care. For this we need information about disease outcomes.

Commissioners of health care will only wish to fund clinical
rheumatology services if they provide continuing evidence that they
are effective by evaluating how they influence clinical outcomes.
Clinical practice in rheumatology must be based on research and
development that will identify effective therapies, determine how to
measure the results of treatment, and defined optimal and likely
outcomes of current treatment. Rheumatoid arthritis is the disease
to use as a template for such work because it is: a common
rheumatic disorder; is managed by all rheumatologists; and is a
clear specialist responsibility.

There is good evidence of the effectiveness of current anti-
rheumatic drugs such as gold and other slow-acting drugs from
individual randomised controlled trial and meta-analyses of trials
of slow-acting drugs. Despite the apparent effectiveness of slow-acting drugs information on disease outcomes in rheumatoid arthritis
from prospective long-term clinical studies show: patients treated
for 10–20 years have poor results with over 80% of cases first seen
as inpatients moderately or severely incapacitated by 20 years; and
the average outpatient has a 30% chance of severe disability. There
are areas of controversy as some studies in early disease suggest a
milder course.

Traditional research into disease mechanisms, epidemiology and
clinical trials should therefore be supplemented by research into
how an optimal clinical rheumatology service can improve disease
outcome. This requires a national collaborative strategy to optimise successful research in this area and avoid unnecessary reduplication of effort. Rheumatologists provide symptomatic help for
most patients with rheumatoid arthritis, but there is continuing
long-term morbidity and mortality. New therapies under development (eg immunotherapy) may improve outcome but will be
expensive and only purchased if their effectiveness and benefits
can be demonstrated.

The first step is to collect simple information relevant to disease
outcomes in routine clinical practice. There is no agreed minimum data set for this purpose. But the health assessment questionnaire, together with details of age, sex, disease duration, treatment

and possibly some measure of disease activity, is likely to be adequate as a first step. At the same time we also need to recognise that there is a cost to collecting even this simple data in routine clinical practice, and it is not inconsiderable. But it is preferable to know the value of treatment than have too much concern about the cost of gaining this information.

7 | Measuring impairment

David L Scott
Reader in Rheumatology, Department of Rheumatology,
King's College Hospital, London

Background

Gradual progression of joint damage is characteristic of rheumatoid arthritis. This is accompanied by increasing deformities and declining function. The evidence suggests structural joint damage is the predominant cause of functional impairment. Structural changes of joints are evaluated by imaging methods. There are associated progressive radiological abnormalities, and it is straightforward to assume that joint radiology gives a good indication of the progression of rheumatoid arthritis and its related functional outcome. For this reason X-rays have been given a central place in assessment of the progression of rheumatoid arthritis. Newer imaging technologies such as magnetic resonance imaging may eventually replace them. There is evidence that MRI is best in early disease and X-rays are better when there are significant bony changes. The use of X-ray in the assessment of disease progression in rheumatoid arthritis depends on three questions: how precisely does radiology reflect joint dynamics, the actual disruption of cartilage and peri-articular bone? What is the best index of the disease progression? How does it relate to X-ray measurements?

Current X-ray scoring methods

These are predominantly those of Sharp *et al* (1971) and Larsen *et al* (1977). Both methods are reproducible (Sharp *et al*, 1985; Grindulis *et al*, 1983). Sharp's method is more sensitive to change (Cuchacovich *et al*, 1992). The scores are composite indices combining joint space loss, erosions and other changes. They have highlighted the value of standardisation. But they combine diverse changes in a single score and assign numerical values to qualitative changes. The 1993 WHO/ILAR Task Force Meeting recommended developing a new approach based on juxta-articular erosions and joint destruction. Until new methods are developed and evaluated the Sharp and Larsen scores should be used.

Prospective randomised studies of anti-rheumatic drugs on X-ray progression

A major debate exists in clinical rheumatology about the long-term effects of slow-acting anti-rheumatic drugs (SAARDS) and whether they influence the progression of the disease. If X-rays allow assessment of the progression of rheumatoid arthritis they can be used to define the long term therapeutic influences on rheumatoid arthritis. This is the second main reason why joint radiology is of interest to follow rheumatoid arthritis patients.

Early placebo controlled studies show reduced radiological progression with gold (Co-operating Clinics Committee, 1973; Sigler *et al*, 1974) and cyclophosphamide (Co-operating Clinics Committee, 1970). Recent work shows sulphasalazine also reduces radiological progression (van der Heijde *et al*, 1989). But several large studies of injectable gold, penicillamine and similar drugs failed to detect effects on X-ray progression. In general studies have been too small, too brief, evaluated only patients remaining on specific therapies, and used too many different methods to determine joint damage.

Observational studies of X-ray progression

X-ray changes in hands and wrists reflect major joints (Scott *et al*, 1985a). In early rheumatoid arthritis 70% of patients have radiological damage at 3 years (van der Heidje *et al*, 1992). By 10 years X-ray progression is invariable in severe disease (Scott *et al*, 1986). By 20 years most of patients have extensive progression despite therapy (Scott *et al*, 1987).

Technical advances and new approaches to measuring progression

Digital image analysis of standard radiographs theoretically increases sensitivity of measurement, but has limited value for assessing erosions (Richmond *et al*, 1992). Microfocal radiology increases sensitivity (Dacre and Buckland-Wright, 1992). The specialised equipment and technical support needed will not become widely available, making it unsuitable as a standard method. Magnetic resonance imaging (MRI) is an area of rapid advance. It is likely to be the dominant method of joint imaging in the next decade (Corvetta *et al*, 1992). Developing new approaches to assessing erosions and joint destruction in rheumatoid arthritis must incorporate concepts from MRI and allow for the probable predominance of MRI techniques.

X-ray measures in future clinical studies

Future clinical studies of anti-rheumatic drugs involving the assessment of prevention or significant decrease in the rate of progression of structural joint damage in rheumatoid arthritis should meet several standards. This view is related to the concept of disease controlling anti-rheumatic therapies (DC-ARTs) which were defined though meetings of the WHO and International League Against Rheumatism (Edmonds *et al*, 1993a, 1993b). This concept and the associated measures which should be taken are summarised in Tables 1–3. All patients entered into a study must be assessed at its completion and not only those who remain on medication. Studies require sufficient power to determine realistic differences due to therapy. They should last long enough for a reliable analysis of the effects of joint damage to be ascertained; 1 year would be the

Table 1. Proposals for studies looking at DC-ART status

1. All patients entered must be assessed on completion
2. Studies must have sufficient power
3. Studies must be long enough - one year is minimum
4. Studies should evaluate erosions in juxta-articular bone
5. Changes in the hands and wrists should be used to indicate overall progression

WHO/ILAR Task Force Meeting, Geneva 1993 (Edmonds *et al*, 1993a, b).

Table 2. Therapeutic aims for DC-ART status

1. Preventing new erosions in early disease
    (<2 years from diagnosis)
2. Preventing new erosions in established disease
    (2–5 years from diagnosis)
3. Reducing the rate erosions develop in established disease
    (<5 years from diagnosis)
4. Reducing the rate of joint destruction in late disease
    (>5 years from diagnosis).

Table 3. Further developmental work on X-rays

1. To define precisely what constitutes erosions and destroyed joints
2. To determine agreement between experienced specialists
3. To quantify the development of erosive damage in different stages of RA
4. To develop a standardised statistical approach for analysis

minimal period of time for such a study, and 2 years would be preferable. Evaluation should concentrate on erosions and related structural changes in juxta-articular bone; mapping osteoporotic areas in early disease may be a sensitive and objective measure. Assessments ought to use changes within the hands and wrists to indicate overall progression, with the feet included in evaluating early disease. There should be different therapeutic aims at various stages of rheumatoid arthritis, focusing on preventing new erosions developing in early disease (<2 years from diagnosis), preventing new erosions occurring in established disease (2–5 years from diagnosis), and both reducing the rate erosions develop in established disease (<5 years from diagnosis) and also reducing the rate of joint destruction in late disease (>5 years from diagnosis).

Surrogate biochemical markers

Although X-rays provide information about bony changes and loss of joint space (and thus the associated cartilage loss in rheumatoid arthritis joints), most of the research into the mechanisms of damage to rheumatoid arthritis joints has concentrated upon cartilage damage alone. A variety of *in vitro* models have shown that two degradative pathways may operate upon articular cartilage simultaneously in rheumatoid arthritis: direct invasion by the rheumatoid arthritis synovial membrane at the marginal pannus; and release of regulatory peptides such as interleukin-1 which act on chondrocytes and cells of the synovium (Arend and Dayer, 1990). While most of these effects are probably mediated by collagenase and other enzymes in the collagenase super-gene family (Murphy and Docherty, 1988) there is a balance between the synthesis of matrix components and their degradation, and some of the changes in the rheumatoid synovium and the associated articular cartilage can be explained by decreased matrix synthesis.

The balance of evidence suggests that the mediators found in rheumatoid arthritis joints will cause persistent inflammation and lead to cartilage damage. Despite these findings there are some doubts about a precise relationship between synovial inflammation and cartilage damage in rheumatoid arthritis, and it has been suggested these may be parallel processes with somewhat different controlling factors (Dayer, 1990).

Many studies have shown that SAARDS affect those mediators which are likely to cause cartilage damage and hence radiological changes in rheumatoid arthritis. For instance, there are several investigations which show that SAARDS such as auranofin, penicillamine and methotrexate influence the production and effects of interleukin-1 and metalloproteinases (Hunneyball *et al*, 1988; Hunter *et al*, 1984; Matsubara and Hirohata, 1988; Remvig *et al*, 1988; Segal *et al*, 1989). The most compelling logic for assuming SAARDS will influence radiological progression comes from studies of the acute phase response. Active rheumatoid arthritis is characterised by a number of acute phase protein changes with an elevated ESR, a high C-reactive protein level, and associated changes in other plasma proteins such as orosomucoid and immunoglobulins (McConkey *et al*, 1980). SAARDs invariably reduce the elevated acute phase response when given to groups of patients with active rheumatoid arthritis, and indeed this is one basis for recognising drugs in this class (Amos *et al*, 1977). There is also considerable evidence that patients with a persistently elevated acute phase response have more radiological progression of their rheumatoid arthritis (Dawes *et al*, 1986). The implication of these observations is that SAARDS should reduce the rate of radiological progression in rheumatoid arthritis, and this was suggested by McConkey and his colleagues from their observations of the effects of SAARD on the acute phase response and on X-ray changes in rheumatoid arthritis patients (Segal *et al*, 1989).

However, the picture is not clear cut. Depending upon the way in which a study is designed it is possible to conclude that either SAARDS reduce the elevated ESR and slow radiological progression in rheumatoid arthritis, or that only the ESR is effectively reduced while X-ray progression continues (Scott *et al*, 1984, 1985b; Pullar and Capell, 1986). This area was extensively investigated in the 1980s and it is unlikely that looking at the interrelationships in greater detail will help to better define the effects of SAARDS on radiological progression.

Bone markers such as assays for pyridinium cross-links (pyridinoline and deoxypyridinoline) and for collagen fragments (collagen I and III propeptides) have yet to be established as important markers in rheumatoid arthritis.

8 | Measuring functional status

Ray Fitzpatrick
Fellow, Nuffield College, Oxford University Lecturer, Department of Public Health and Primary Care, University of Oxford

Introduction

This chapter is concerned with a range of measures that may be used to assess outcomes in rheumatoid arthritis (RA) in terms of the patient's perspective. These measures are referred to in the literature by a variety of terms which include 'functional status', 'health status' and 'health-related quality of life' measures. All of the instruments discussed in this chapter are in questionnaire format and can be completed by patients without assistance. The desirable measurement properties of such questionnaires are now well established and familiar (Fitzpatrick *et al*, 1992). They should be *reliable* in the sense of yielding the same results on repeated uses under the same conditions; *valid* in that they measure what they purport to measure and *responsive* in that they are capable of detecting significant changes over time. Validity in particular is difficult to establish when there are no 'gold standards' against which to measure what is by definition a personal and subjective phenomenon. However, a variety of ways have now been developed to enhance the validity of a questionnaire. Questionnaires in this field should, as far as possible, be developed from patients' own concerns and priorities, rather those of professionals or researchers. Their content validity is examined informally by inspecting whether questionnaire items adequately cover issues of concern. Construct validity is examined with reference to more formal evidence of relationships of the new instrument to other information such as disease stage and severity.

Context and purpose of measurement

In addition to the three formal psychometric criteria for assessing measures of functional status in RA, there are, under the real world constraints of either individual patient care or clinical trials, more informal but equally important requirements. Instruments need to be acceptable to patients, practically feasible (both in terms of completion by patients and subsequent data processing) and relevant to the particular problem or issue at hand. Thus it is important to examine closely the particular context of use to which an instrument is going to be put. A functional status instrument might be used to 'screen' for functional problems in an out-patient clinic in which case the range of aspects of function it assesses would be particularly important together with the ability to discriminate between levels of function between patients at a point in time. In a clinical trial a greater emphasis would be placed on the ability of an instrument to pick up possibly subtle but still significant changes over time within patients. In the former context construct validity is of greater concern; in the latter responsiveness. The specific use to which an instrument is to be put is also relevant when considering validity. It is important to understand that no instrument is ever valid *tout court*; it is valid for those applications in which it has actually been tested.

Range of available measures

Rheumatology is one of the health care specialties, alongside oncology and cardiology, relatively well endowed with health status instruments. For the most part they have been used in research contexts and there is far less evidence regarding their applicability to other contexts such as quality assurance, evaluation or individual patient care. The two most familiar instruments for use in arthritis are the Health Assessment Questionnaire (HAQ) (Fries *et al*, 1982) and the Arthritis Impact Measurement Scales (AIMS) (Meenan *et al*, 1980). Other instruments developed for use in RA include the Lee Functional Index (Lee *et al*, 1973) the Toronto Activities of Daily Living Questionnaire (Helewa *et al*, 1982), the McMaster Health Index Questionnaire (MHIQ) (Chambers *et al*, 1982), and the MACTAR Patient Preference Disability Questionnaire (Tugwell *et al*, 1987). However, only the HAQ and AIMS from this list have received sufficiently widespread attention that it is possible to assess their potential value.

In addition to instruments developed specifically for use in RA (so-called 'disease-specific' measures), there are now several questionnaires that have been designed to be relevant to a wide range of health problems (so called 'generic' measures). A number of such generic instruments have been used to assess health status in

RA, including the Sickness Impact Profile (SIP) (Deyo *et al*, 1982); the Nottingham Health Profile (NHP) (Hunt *et al*, 1985); the Quality of Well-Being Scale (QWB) (Balaban *et al*, 1986); the Functional Status Questionnaire (FSQ) (Jette *et al*, 1986); The Farmer Quality of Life Scale (Rudick *et al*, 1992); the SF-36 (Ware, 1993).

It is important to recognise that although all of the instruments cited above have been used in assessing functional status in RA and generally appear to have rather similar range and content, they may produce different evidence regarding patients' well being. Thus, in one study patients with RA were asked to complete one disease-specific instrument (AIMS) and one generic instrument (NHP) on two occasions 3 months apart (Fitzpatrick *et al*, 1991). Patients' scores in relation to mobility agreed quite substantially for the two instruments. There was somewhat less agreement regarding scores for emotional distress. Most strikingly patients' scores with regard to social function did not correlate significantly. For emotional and social function, the two health status instruments gave quite substantially different pictures of patients' well-being.

Short-term outcomes

Health status measures in RA need to play a role with regard to both short-term and longer- term changes in RA. Far more evidence is available about the performance of health status measures in the short term (2 years or less), whereas given the long-term course of overall deterioration in disability in RA, it is equally important to have evidence of the performance of health status measures over much longer periods (10 years or longer).

With regard to short-term changes many of the health status measures reviewed above have been shown to have some satisfactory measurement properties in terms of reliability, validity and responsiveness to change in relation to RA. Recent reviews provide evidence of satisfactory measurement properties of the HAQ, AIMS, SIP, NHP, MHIQ, FSQ (Guccione and Jette, 1990; Fitzpatrick, 1993). The most striking evidence of the value of functional status measures is to be found in several randomised controlled trials (RCTs) in which patient-based measures have identified differences between effective therapies and placebo. The HAQ in particular has proved sensitive to significant clinical changes in RA in a number of trials. Significant improvement in RA were shown over a 6 month period on HAQ disability scores for patients treated with auranofin compared with placebo (Bombardier *et al*,

1986). A 24 month double blind trial also showed significant benefits of auranofin for HaQ disability scores (Borg *et al*, 1988). The
HAQ has also proved to be sensitive to improvements in disability
in RA produced by psycho-educational interventions (Mullen *et al*,
1987).

The AIMS has also been included in several RCTs. Oral and
injectable gold were compared with placebo over a 21 week trial
(Meenan *et al*, 1984). Significant differences between active drugs
and placebo were found for pain and psychological but not physical dimensions of AIMS. In another trial diclofenac was compared
with aspirin or naproxen over a 12 week period (Anderson *et al*,
1989). The study drug produced significantly more favourable
results for physical, pain and psychological dimensions of AIMS.
Indeed much of the improvement related to the study drug was
visible within 4 weeks of entry to the trial.

Although other instruments such as the SIP (Ahlmen *et al*, 1988)
and the Quality of Well-Being Scale (Bombardier *et al*, 1991) are
beginning to be used as outcome measures in RCTs so that evidence of their responsiveness can be assessed, at present there is
far more evidence to support the responsiveness of the HAQ than
exists for other measures.

Longer-term outcomes

RA is a chronic disease and requires follow-up over 20 years or
more fully to assess the course of disease and outcomes of treatment. Unfortunately we know very little about the longer-term performance of health status measures in RA as only studies using the
HAQ or variants of HAQ have been reported. The most extensive
study is of a series of 1,274 patients with RA who attended a private
rheumatology practice in Wichita, Kansas for up to 12 years (Wolfe
and Cathey, 1991). The study produces clear evidence of progressive deterioration in disability. Thus they estimate that half of
patients with RA will reach a score of 2.5 on HAQ (equivalent to
very severe disability) 10 years after their first clinic visit. Another
study is reported of 330 individuals who volunteered for a study of
RA in California and were followed up over 8 years (Leigh and
Fries, 1992). This study also obtained evidence of progressive deterioration as measured by HAQ scores although not as marked as
the rate of deterioration in the Kansas sample. It is not clear
whether this is due to the fact that Kansas patients had more severe
histories because of clinic rather than community recruitment.

Leigh and Fries (1992) note that in their longitudinal series those patients with the most severe HAQ scores at the beginning of the study experienced less subsequent deterioration than individuals with initially more favourable scores. They suggest that one possibility for this is that patients may reach a 'plateau' in their disease. However, another possibility that needs to be considered is that the HAQ may be subject to 'ceiling' effects of a kind noted for other health status measures (Bindman *et al,* 1990). This term refers to the possibility that a health status instrument may be incapable of registering the deterioration that occurs in patients beyond the poorest scores recognised by the instrument. There is evidence to suggest that, over the longer term, HAQ may be prone to ceiling effects. Gardiner *et al* (1993) administered the HAQ to 245 RA inpatients and outpatients at the beginning and end of a 5 year period. They noted overall deterioration in HAQ scores as had the studies of RA in Kansas and California samples. However, when subgroups in terms of baseline HAQ scores were analysed, those patients with the poorest initial scores tended, 5 years later, to rate their RA as 'worse' or 'much worse'. However, this group experienced no mean change score for HAQ over the 5 year period. By comparison other groups with more favourable initial HAQ scores, who viewed their RA as having deteriorated to a smaller extent, registered *larger* amounts of deterioration in 5 year HAQ scores. The most plausible explanation for these results is the one offered by Gardiner *et al* (1993), that deterioration at the extreme levels of disability may be undetected by HAQ because of ceiling effects.

Comparative studies of instruments

So many are the available health status measures of relevance to RA that, in recent years studies have begun directly to compare the performance of different instruments. The design of such studies requires that patients complete several instruments at various points over time and the sensitivity to change of instruments are then directly compared. Some external evidence that change has truly occurred is required; either that patients have experienced an effective medical or surgical intervention or that they judge their health to have improved or declined. Liang *et al* (1984) compared the performance of five health status instruments (AIMS, FSI, SIP, HAQ, QWB) in patients with either RA or osteoarthritis before and 3 months after hip or knee replacement surgery. Change scores were compared for comparable dimensions of the five instruments: pain, mobility, social function and global scores.

The HAQ was somewhat less sensitive to changes in pain and mobility than other instruments. The AIMS was somewhat less sensitive in the assessment of social function compared to other instruments. However, overall no instrument was consistently more sensitive to changes, and in particular, no consistent differences were noted between generic instruments and those developed specifically for use in arthritis. In a subsequent paper Liang *et al* (1990) examined changes between preoperative state and one year later for the same sample. Broadly the same trends were noted as for short-term outcomes. The same group (Katz *et al*, 1992) have reported another comparative study on OA and RA patients undergoing hip replacement surgery. A different group of health status measures were examined. The main conclusion of this study was that shorter instruments such as SF-36 seemed just as sensitive to changes over time as longer instruments such as the SIP.

A few comparative studies of health status measures have also been carried out with patients with RA receiving medical rather than surgical care. Patients receiving medical treatments are an important group in which to compare the performance of instruments because changes tend to be more subtle and more difficult to detect. In a RCT of auranofin compared with placebo, a number of different types of instrument were also compared (Bombardier *et al*, 1991). In the measurement of pain, a simple visual analogue line appeared slightly more sensitive to change than either a ten point pain 'ladder' or the quite detailed McGill Pain Questionnaire (Melzack, 1975). In the assessment of functional status, the HAQ appeared slightly less sensitive than the QWB questionnaire. Of all the clinical, laboratory, radiological and health status measures used, the measure that proved most sensitive to differences between active and placebo drug was a simple five point scale to rate their RA ('very poor' to 'very good') completed by the patient and developed specifically for the study.

In a comparative study of change scores for the HAQ and SIP over a 15 month period, both instruments appeared similarly sensitive to changes in patients as assessed by the clinician or according to the Mallya and Mace Index (Fitzpatrick *et al*, 1989). However, it might be argued that the criteria against which to compare instruments should be the patient's own judgement of whether a significant change for better or worse has occurred. In accordance with this view a study was conducted in which patients completed four health status instruments (AIMS, HAQ, SIP, NHP) every 3 months (Fitzpatrick *et al*, 1993a). They also reported their views of change in response to 'transition questions' in which patients rated their current RA compared with a previous occasion on a five point scale (from 'very much worse' to 'very much better'). It was thus possible to compare change scores between two time periods for different instruments amongst a homogeneous subgroup of the sample who all viewed their RA as, for example, improved. Overall instruments performed rather similarly, and there was no evidence of longer instruments or instruments developed specifically for RA being more sensitive to the changes emphasised by patients in transition questions. Some subscales of the AIMS, particularly Household Activity, Activities of Daily Living (ADL) and Social scales, appeared insensitive to change. Other evidence also indicated insensitivity of the AIMS ADL scale in mildly impaired patients (Potts and Brandt, 1987). Overall similarities in performance of SIP and AIMS are supported in another comparative study of patients with OA (Weinberger *et al*, 1992).

In summary, whilst in some comparative studies particular instruments appear to have scales or dimensions that are more or less sensitive than others, the most striking overall feature of the available evidence from the short-term comparative studies so far carried out is that no single instrument dominates others in sensitivity to change. Moreover, shorter instruments may be as sensitive as longer instruments to important changes. If this is the case then instruments may well be selected in terms of other criteria such as length of time required for patients to complete the questionnaire and investigators to process the information. By this criterion the HAQ has considerable advantages as the shortest of the instruments discussed in this review. The HAQ may take as little as 3 to 5 minutes to complete and 20 seconds to score (Wolfe *et al*, 1988). Other instruments have not been systematically timed but are almost certain to require more time overall to process.

Patients' personal priorities

A number of recent developments in functional status measurement have been intended to make questionnaires more personally relevant to individual respondents. Thus O'Boyle and colleagues (1992) have developed an interview schedule—the Schedule for the Evaluation of Individual Quality of Life (SEIQoL) which elicits patients' five personally identified priorities in life and the personal weight or importance attached to identified priorities. This detailed instrument has been used to assess patients' quality of life before and after hip replacement surgery. The instrument identified improvements in quality of life 6 months after surgery.

However, change scores for SEIQoL were not as substantial as for two more conventional, standardised instruments, the AIMS and MHIQ. This would not appear to be a method that is very practical in its current form, as it requires skilled and time-consuming interviewing and substantial processing and analysis of results. A somewhat simpler approach which also attempts to identify individuals' priorities is the MACTAR questionnaire developed by Tugwell *et al* (1987). Individuals with RA are asked to identify up to five activities adversely affected by RA and then to rank order their nominated activities as priorities or preferences. Patients are on subsequent occasions asked to rate whether changes have occurred in ability to pursue nominated activities. In an 8 week study with 50 patients, change scores for personally expressed preferences were more sensitive than a conventional standardised questionnaire against the criterion of a global question of change in RA. This methodology was further tested in a controlled trial of methotrexate in which outcomes were assessed in terms of the MACTAR measures of individualised preferences and a conventional health status instrument. The MACTAR instrument produced greater differences in change scores between active treatment and placebo than did the conventional health status questionnaire (Tugwell *et al*, 1990). Although such methods would appear to be particularly sensitive to patients' priorities and are quite appropriate as measures of outcome, it is not yet clear that they can be used routinely in a clinical context as they require sensitive interviewing to be properly conducted.

Transition questions

Another way in which patients' experiences of outcome can be more directly elicited is by means of 'transition questions' in which they are invited directly to judge whether any important change (for better or worse) has occurred since a specific previous occasion. The Modified HAQ (Pincus *et al*, 1983) contains such transition questions in relation to eight areas of disability. To assess the value of this form of question, patients were asked to complete the HAQ on two occasions 3 months apart and change scores were calculated from the differences between scores (Ziebland *et al*, 1992). On the second assessment patients also completed the transition items of the Modified HAQ. These transition data correlated considerably more strongly with various other standard rheumatological measures of change than did change scores on the conventional HAQ. It was inferred that patients observe significant degrees of change in disability that may be detected by the conventional HAQ. Even a single global transition question asking patients to rate overall effects of RA compared to a previous occasion on a five point scale (from 'much better' to 'much worse'), has substantial validity, correlating with change scores for a wide range of clinical, laboratory and health status measures (Fitzpatrick *et al*, 1993b). It is not clear whether such judgements can play a role in relation to longer-term changes in RA, but, in formats such as the Modified HAQ they offer a simple and informative form of short-term patient-based outcome measure.

General Comments

Although substantial progress has been made in the development of measures to assess outcomes of RA from the patient's perspective, it is just as important to develop instruments that will actually be used in clinical practice. Ultimately as with any other screening, diagnostic or evaluative device, use of health status measures must improve the quality of care. Kazis *et al* (1990) carried out a detailed study to investigate the usefulness of health status reports in RA. A sample of 1,920 patients with RA in various community practices in Boston and Nashville were randomised to one of three groups. In the study group they completed either the AIMS or Modified HAQ on a quarterly basis over a year and results were processed and sent to their doctor. In an 'attention placebo' group patients completed a health status measure on the same basis but results were not sent to their doctor. A third 'placebo' group only completed health status measures at the beginning and end of the year. The study examined whether giving doctors health status data would alter either *how* they treated patients or the outcomes of care. There were no detectable differences in any measures, such as medication compliance, numbers of visits to the doctor or of referrals to other services, patient satisfaction or health status, despite the fact that a majority of doctors reported finding the receipt of health status data helpful. These are disappointing results. They may have arisen because doctors did not receive the health status data at times that coincided with patients' visits. It may also be that one year is too short a timeframe for the study. Nevertheless the study underlines the need to evaluate health status measures in terms of practical uses to which they may be put.

  In summary, no measure to date fulfils all of the criteria whereby we judge health status measures. More work is needed to evaluate the role and value of measures in this field. The HAQ has to date received far more attention than other instruments and in many respects stands up well as a measure of functional status. It also has the merits of being quite short and lending itself to quite simple processing and intuitively accessible results. Despite certain limitations discussed in the course of the chapter, no other instrument at present consistently 'out-performs' the HAQ. It is increasingly clear that shorter instruments, as well as being more readily processed, may actually be as sensitive to important aspects of health status and changes in health status as longer and more detailed measures. Especially for shorter-term monitoring of patients the HAQ would appear to be highly appropriate as a measure of functional status.

9 | Measuring handicap

Alison J Carr
Research Associate, Department of Social Medicine,
University of Bristol

Introduction

Rheumatoid arthritis (RA) is a chronic disease of unknown aetiology and unpredictable course and prognosis. It is associated with significant levels of pain (Callahan *et al*, 1987; Kazis *et al*, 1983) and functional disability (Yelin *et al*, 1987; Tugwell *et al*, 1987) and has a wider psychosocial impact on exercise and recreation (Deyo *et al*, 1982; Yelin *et al*, 1987), relationships (Liang *et al*, 1984; Masters *et al*, 1983), psychological well-being (Bishop *et al*, 1987; Frank *et al*, 1988) and ability to work (Meenan *et al*, 1981; Yelin *et al*, 1980). It therefore has a major impact in many areas of individuals' lives not traditionally considered the domain of medical intervention. Given the current inability of medicine to prevent or cure RA, the primary aim of medical care is a reduction in the impact of RA. This has led to calls for the focus of health care to be on the quality, rather than the duration, of life (Fries, 1980) with a postponement of the disabling effects of RA being one of the major treatment objectives. To this end, measures are required to identify and assess the disabling consequences of RA and the effectiveness of medical attempts to prevent or postpone them.

In acknowledgement of the wider psychosocial consequences of chronic disease, and in an attempt to distinguish between the clinical and social consequences, the World Health Organisation (WHO, 1980) provided definitions of impairment, disability and handicap (Table 1). The measurement of impairment in RA is synonymous with the measurement of disease activity and is well established. Measures of disability, in the guise of physical function, have been used in RA since 1937 (Taylor, 1937) and have become increasingly sophisticated over time. The search for some measure which incorporates some of the broader aspects of health and consequences of disease has led to an upsurge of interest in

Table 1. World Health Organisation definitions of impairment, disability and handicap (WHO, 1980)

Impairment	Any loss or abnormality of psychological or anatomical structure or function
Disability	Any restriction or lack (resulting from impairment) of ability to perform an activity in the manner or within the range considered normal for a human being
Handicap	A disadvantage for an individual resulting from impairment or disability that limits or prevents the fulfilment of a role that is normal (depending on age, sex and cultural factors) for that individual

generic quality of life measures. Whilst their attempts to identify and quantify consequences of disease important to patients are laudable, their usefulness is limited by the problems of interpretation; a quality of life measure would give the clinician an overall impression of how much impact disease has on an individual but would not enable him to identify specific problems which may be amenable to treatment or intervention of some kind. According to the WHO definitions of disease impact, the dimension missing in current assessments is the disadvantage suffered by an individual as a result of disease, ie handicap.

What is handicap?

Handicap, the social consequence of disease, is specific to individuals and depends not only on the severity of disease, but also on his or her life role. The latter is itself dependent on many factors including physical and psychological make-up, expectations of family and society and individual aspirations. This means that the same impairment can result in different handicaps and handicaps of varying severity. For example, a young patient may suffer painful hand deformity (impairment) rendering her unable to write (disability), leading to the loss of her job as a secretary (handicap). However, for an 80 year old woman, the same impairment and disability may mean that she becomes socially isolated because she is unable to write to her friends, or get dressed to go out to meet them. The degree to which an individual is handicapped depends on the perception of the importance of the role that can no longer be filled. Thus the degree to which the young secretary was handicapped by losing her job might be different if she was a single parent or living with her employed husband.

Handicaps can be defined with reference to either society's or the individual's perspective and discrepancies between the two views can be considerable. Society, in the guise of employers and health care professionals among others, defines individuals as handicapped or disadvantaged when they are unable to fulfil roles which someone of a similar age, sex and social background would be expected to perform. This assessment takes no account of the individual's aspirations and expectations. For example, a keen amateur musician with relatively mild rheumatoid arthritis may find that he is unable to play his instrument, but is able to continue work as a personnel manager. In societal terms, he would not be considered handicapped, but at a personal level, the loss of what is to him a very important activity would represent considerable disadvantage. Both views are valid but suited to different situations. In epidemiological or population studies, some comparison with a defined norm is useful and the use of society-perceived measures of handicap would be appropriate. At a clinical level, however, assessment of the individual's perception of the impact of disease and the particular problems which he/she experiences is more relevant.

Why is assessment of handicap important?

Firstly, it is often possible to alleviate handicap, even when impairment and disability seem insurmountable. For example, the inability to walk outdoors may not be amenable to change, but the resultant handicap (being housebound) may be alleviated by the use of a wheelchair.

The measurement of patient-perceived handicap in chronic disease would provide the clinician with information about the meaning of disease for each individual patient and would enable treatment and intervention to be tailored to meet each individual patient's needs. In some cases, the handicaps which have been identified may require treatments or interventions which are difficult to provide because of resource restrictions (for example, clinical psychology). In these cases, the identification of a number of patients requiring the same intervention will lend weight to applications for that resource. Identified handicaps may also result in the development of new interventions, such as a programme to help people develop a more positive body image.

Measuring patient-perceived handicap would provide clinically relevant information which could not be collected by biological measures of disease activity or functional disability questionnaires. For example, an increase in reported pain and disease activity in someone with RA may be the result of a major life event such as a bereavement or loss of employment (Fifield *et al*, 1991) and this information is important for the appropriate management of that individual.

On a more global level, the concept of handicap can act as an agent for political and social change. In many countries people with disabilities are socially disadvantaged because of societal prejudice. The remedy in this situation is a change in society, rather than the individual. In this instance, adoption of the concept of handicap is necessary to allow planners and politicians to address society's responsibility. One example of a situation where this theory has been put into practice is in a community-based rehabilitation programme in Pakistan where a handicap scale has been used to identify training needs among disabled people (Finnstam *et al*, 1988).

Models of disease and illness: the relationship between impairment, disability and Handicap

At first sight it might be anticipated that the relationship between impairment, disability and handicap is hierarchical (Fig. 1) as implied by the WHO model. Thus, the greater the joint damage, the less able an individual will be to undertake a specific task and consequently the more disadvantaged. However, in RA this is not the case. In 1974 De Haas and colleagues described a group of patients who functioned normally despite severe, nodular, seropositive RA (De Haas *et al*, 1974). Similarly, there have been reports of higher disability scores in women compared with men with similar severity and duration of RA (Thompson and Pegley, 1991). Conversely, practising rheumatologists are familiar with the patient with mild, inactive RA who seems inappropriately crippled by their disease. These observations support the contention that factors other than the disease process are important in determining the impact of the disease on an individual.

Other models of disablement have been proposed which incorporate the influence of these factors. The Situational Handicap Model (Minaire, 1983) depicts disablement as a social system functioning in a given environment and exchanging permanently and regularly with both the cultural and biophysical components of the environment. It separates situational disablement into three distinct constituents: the individual biomedical, psychological and social process, the disabling situations experienced by the person or group, and the environment of the system, encompassing the

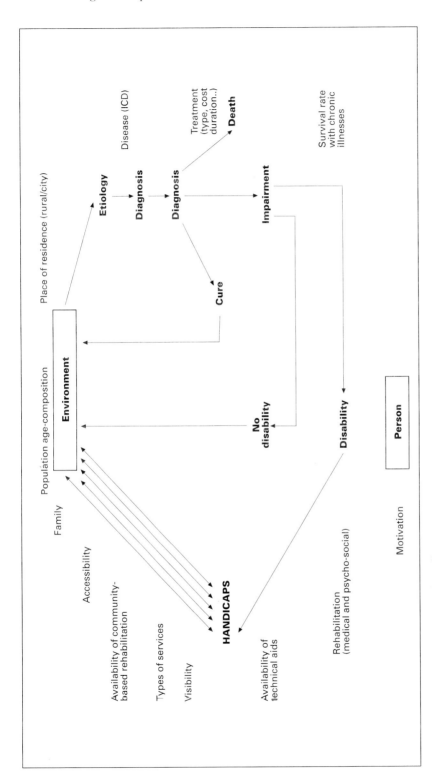

Fig 1. A hierarchical model of handicap

cultural, ecological, physical, economic, legal, religious and other factors. Situational disablement is said to occur when there is an imbalance between individual, situational and environmental inputs and outputs. One danger with this model is that reducing the process of disablement exclusively to a situational experience ignores the biomedical and psychological history of the individual. In practical terms this can lead to problems if the model is used to plan and implement the social treatment of handicap.

In an attempt to counteract the deficiencies inherent in both models and to operationalise the concepts to facilitate assessment, a unifying schema of the disablement process has been proposed (Fig 2) (Minaire, 1992). The result is a comprehensive but complex model which, despite acknowledging the influence of environmental, social and cultural factors on the experience of handicap, still adheres to the concept of a linear relationship between impairment, disability and handicap.

An examination of clinical situations already described undermines the validity of a linear relationship. Clinical experience, particularly in the field of dermatology, indicates that handicap, usually social disadvantage as a result of the disfiguring aspects of some dermatological conditions, can occur in patients who are not disabled. In these cases, the impairment has been the direct cause of handicap. The relationship between impairment, disability and handicap might therefore be better represented by a Venn diagram (Fig 3) (Carr and Thompson, 1994b).

The importance of understanding the relationships between the disease processes and the effect of those processes on an individual becomes paramount when considering treatment. If the relationship was hierarchical then an approach concentrating on control

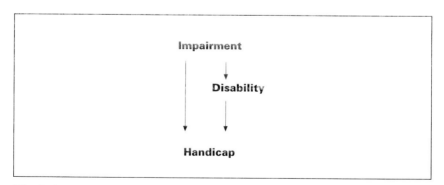

Fig 2. A unifying schema of impairment, disability and handicap. From Minnaire (1992)

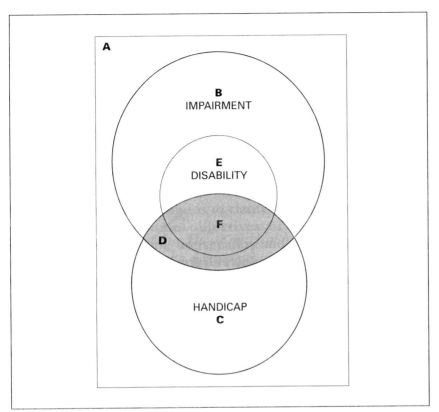

Fig 3. Venn diagram depicting an interactive, multidimensional relationship between impairment, disability and handicap. The Venn diagram illustrates the relationship between impairment, disability and handicap as it occurs in the general population. The majority of people do not experience impairment, disability or handicap (area A). Some people have impairments but no disabilities or handicaps (area B), for example people who have evidence of osteoarthritis on X-ray but are asymptomatic. Others are handicapped without having impairments or disabilities ie not health-related handicap (area C). An example would be people who are unemployed for reasons unrelated to their health. A number of people have impairments and handicaps without experiencing disabilities (area D), for example a teenage girl with a port wine stain on her face who is socially handicapped. Health-related disabilities only occur when some impairment is present (area E). A proportion of the population experience impairment, disability and handicap (area F). The shaded area represents health-related handicap. From Carr and Thompson (1994b)

of impairments (disease activity, joint damage) would be enough as this would necessarily lead to reduction in disability and handicap. As this is not the case, alternative measures may be necessary to minimise the impact of the disease.

Measuring handicap

The measurement of handicap in chronic disease is in its infancy. There are a few generic tools which purport to measure handicap (Rankin, 1957; Jeffreys *et al*, 1969; Herbert *et al*, 1988; Affleck *et al*, 1988) but these either measure disability rather than handicap, or where they do measure handicap, cover only the physical independence dimension.

The World Health Organisation, in an attempt to provide a classification scheme for the different phases of the consequences of disease which could be used for trial purposes, produced the International Classification of Impairments, Disabilities and Handicaps (ICIDH) (WHO, 1980). This manual contains a series of codes for classifying levels of impairment, disability and handicap. It has been used to assess disabled people in institutional settings (Lankhorst *et al*, 1985; Last, 1985), in population surveys (Colvez and Robine, 1986; de Kleijn-de Vrankrijker, 1986) and for administrative purposes (Hunfield, 1986). In all these situations difficulties have been reported with its use which relate to the exact format of the codes in the classifications and assignment to these codes, the purpose for which it is used and the relationship between impairment, disability and handicap. The handicap scales in particular have proved difficult to use. Experience of the clinical use of the handicap scales indicates that a considerable amount of time is required to gather enough information to allow accurate classification of handicap (Last, 1985; Roy *et al*, 1992). This results in problems with staff cooperation (Roy *et al*, 1992). A further problem, which has implications for the reliability of the classification, is that different professions rate handicap differently (Grimby *et al*, 1988). The general consensus seems to be that while the classification serves a purpose, further development work is needed, particularly with regard to the concept of handicap, to achieve standardisation and agreement about how it should be used.

There are two established instruments which come closer than any others to measuring health-related handicap. The first is a new tool which was designed to measure individual quality of life, the Schedule for the Evaluation of Individual Quality of Life (SEIQoL) (O'Boyle *et al*, 1992). This is an individualised measure of quality of life in which patients are asked by an interviewer to list the five areas of life that they consider to be most important to their overall quality of life. They are then asked to rate their current status in each of these areas on a visual analogue scale (VAS). To quantify the relative weight of each of these areas to the individual's perception of quality of life, they are presented with 30 hypo-thetical people profiles and are asked to rate on a VAS the quality of life they associate with each profile. This tool comes close to measuring the individual handicap resulting from disease but, because it is global rather than specific, and time consuming and expensive to administer, it is a research measure of outcome rather than a clinical tool.

The MACTAR Patient Preference Questionnaire (Tugwell *et al*, 1987) goes some way towards measuring handicap related to func-tional and social activities in that it assesses the disadvantage expe-rienced by individuals in fulfilling roles. Use of the MACTAR as a clinical outcome measure (Tugwell *et al*, 1990) demonstrates the importance of patients' perceptions in assessing the impact of disease.

New handicap measures

An instrument to measure society-perceived handicap in individu-als, the London Health Impact Questionnaire, is currently being developed (Harwood *et al*, 1995). It measures the handicap state of an individual by comparison with the 'normal' activities/lifestyle of someone of a similar age, sex and background who does not have health problems. The disadvantage of the individual in comparison with society determined norms is measured in each of the six survival roles identified by the ICIDH (orientation, physical independence, mobility, occupation, social integration and economic self-sufficiency) and quantified using utilities. This tool will only measure the individual's perception of him/herself as handicapped to the extent that his/her views coincide with those of the general public. It will measure society-perceived handicap and will be of most use as a measure of outcome in between-group comparisons.

A disease specific measure of patient-perceived handicap in RA, the Disease Repercussion Profile, has been developed and validat-ed (Carr and Thompson, 1994a). It produces a profile of per-ceived handicap in six domains, functional activities, social activi-ties, socio-economic status, relationships, emotional well-being and body image using a combination of open questions and graphic rating scales. It is a self-completed questionnaire on which patients are able to specify the particular handicaps they are currently experiencing in each of the domains and rate its severity on a 10 point graphic rating scale. This tool provides an individualised measure of patient-perceived handicap in rheumatoid arthritis. It is quick and easy to complete (10 minutes) and easy to score and interpret. It is currently used routinely in outpatient clinics in one centre and in research projects in a number of others. It is being validated for use in a number of other chronic conditions such as back pain and osteoporosis.

Conclusion

Measuring handicap in rheumatoid arthritis provides important clinical and social information which is missing from existing outcome measures. There is no suggestion that patient-perceived handicap should replace traditional measures of disease activity or functional disability in assessing outcomes in rheumatoid arthritis. However, as an adjunct to these measures, it enables clinicians to treat both the disease and the individual, providing the missing dimension in outcome measurement.

10 | Combined measures and practical issues

Deborah PM Symmons
Consultant Senior Lecturer, ARC Epidemiology Research Unit,
School of Epidemiology and Health Sciences,
University of Manchester

Introduction

The primary considerations when selecting any quantitative measure in clinical medicine are that it should be valid, reliable and feasible. When assessing outcome it is also important to choose measures which are sensitive to change; that is measures which are responsive. In order to be sensitive to change, the measure must both be capable of change in the short term and have a small standard deviation.

Goals of treatment

There are several goals of treatment in rheumatoid arthritis (RA). These aims include the wish to reduce pain and stiffness, to minimise synovitis, to maximise the patient's function and to improve her quality of life. In addition, treatment aims to produce the minimum number of side-effects and to be cost-effective. In order to measure the success or otherwise of therapeutic strategies a different instrument is needed for each of these domains. It would clearly be helpful if everyone used the same outcome measures, so that comparisons between rheumatologists and with published data could be made. As this monograph outlines, there is a choice of instruments for some of the above areas.

Selecting outcome measures

There are established guidelines for selecting outcome measures. They must be valid—that is they must measure what they claim to measure. They must be reliable or reproducible; and they must be feasible in the proposed setting. Many of the valid and reliable measures are not feasible in the routine outpatient setting because they take too long to administer or require complex equipment.

Measures must have the ability to assess progression and be responsive to change. A measure is responsive if it is capable of change. The Steinbrocker functional class (Steinbrocker *et al*, 1949) is not sensitive—it changes very little over long periods of time. If a measure has a large standard deviation (SD) it is impossible to distinguish the change recorded from random error. Walking time and morning stiffness (EMS) have large SDs and so are not sensitive to change.

Pooled indices

Disease outcome in RA is multidimensional and so outcome must be assessed in a number of domains. The situation can appear very confusing if some measures get better while others get worse. There is therefore something inherently appealing about an index which pools several outcome measures and comes up with a single answer. A combined index is composed of a number of measures appropriately selected and weighted. Statistically derived indices have the added advantage of minimising the number of measures included since they select items which are not closely correlated with one another. Increasing the numbers of components in an index can affect its SD. If the components are closely correlated there is no advantage. However, the less well correlated the components the greater will be the fall in SD with the addition of each component—up to about six components. Thus pooled indices are also more sensitive to change because they have a smaller standard deviation than each of the individual items they incorporate. This means that smaller sample sizes are needed in clinical trials in order to demonstrate clinically important differences. Thus a pooled index may be the best single outcome measure in a clinical trial. There are already some pooled indices available. They have been devised in a number of ways, usually either by nominal consensus or statistically. Examples include the disease activity index derived by van der Heijde (1990 and 1992b), the Stoke index (Davis *et al*, 1990), and the Mallya and Mace index (1981). Most are for disease activity alone. In a clinical trial setting then there is much to commend combined measures. However, there are some disadvantages in the routine clinic setting. Pooled indices may be difficult to calculate and to understand and interpret their results.

Overall status measures in RA (OSRA)

In order to overcome these difficulties the rheumatology units at
the Manchester Royal Infirmary and Stoke on Trent have developed an overall status measure in RA(OSRA) for use in the routine
clinic. OSRA has four components: demography, a disease activity
score, a damage score and a treatment category. OSRA uses only
information collected routinely (no blood tests or X-rays), and
takes 30 seconds to compute. The development of the OSRA was
motivated by wanting a measure which could be used in every
patient at every clinic. This would enable, at long last, comparison
of the outcome of routine practice at different centres.

OSRA has four components. The first draws on the three main
demographic factors which influence the prognosis of RA: age,
gender and disease duration. The second and third components
consist of activity and damage scores based on the Apgar score
for newborn babies—in other words each has five items scored 0,
1, 2. For example, for current disease activity the patient is asked
about their well-being (since the last visit), to describe the pain in
the last week, the duration of their morning stiffness, the number
of active joints and the presence of extra-articular disease. None
of these items requires laboratory tests and, for example, the
joint count requires only a rough idea of the number of active
joints. The five areas for the damage score are physical function,
social function, destroyed large and small joints, and organ
impairment due to the disease or its treatment. The fourth component comprises treatment recorded by category (eg non-
steroidals alone; second-line agents plus steroids; cytotoxics). The
components of the OSRA are shown in Table 1 and the scoring
system is shown in the Appendix.

Validity and sensitivity to change

The OSRA has been shown to be valid and reproducible (Symmons *et al*, 1995). It takes less than 30 seconds to complete and
uses standard questions employed in most routine consultations.
The activity score has been shown to correlate with the ESR and C-
reactive protein (CRP). The damage score has been shown to correlate with the health assessment questionnaire (HAQ) and radiological score. In addition, in a cross-sectional study, the damage
score rose with each decade of disease duration. It was evaluated
during 71 inpatient admissions to assess its sensitivity to change.
The activity score improved in the majority of patients. Figure 1

Table 1. Components of the OSRA

1.	Sex: M/F				
	Age: in years				
	Disease duration: A~ <10, B~ 10–20, C~ >20 years				
2.	ACTIVITY	0	1	2	
	Well-being	Same/better	Worse	Much worse	
	Joint pain	None/mild	Moderate	Severe	
	EMS	< 30 min	30–60	> 60	
	Active joint count	< 3	3–10	> 10	
	Extra-articular disease (EAD)	None	New nodules	Vasulitis, serositis, other EAD	
	Total				
3.	DAMAGE				
	Function	Mild	Problems to dress, eat, climb stairs	Housebound	
	Social life	Normal	Moderately impaired	severely impaired	
	Number of destroyed/ replaced large joints	0	1–2	≥ 3	
	Small joint damage	Mild	Needs collar, special shoes, hand splints	Surgery done/needed	
	Organ impairment (> 6/12 months)	None or mild	skin or muscle	Major organ	
	Total				
4.	A. None analgesics steroids B. NSAID alone C. Second-line		D. Second line and E. Cytotoxic ± steroids F. Steroids		
	Summary				

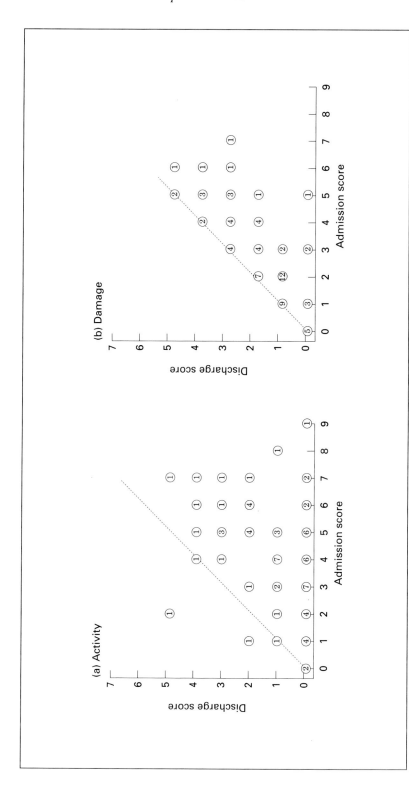

Fig 1. Change in the activity and damage components of the OSRA score during hospital admission for RA. (a) Activity. (b) Damage. Numbers in circles represent numbers of patients. From Symmons *et al*, 1995

illustrates these changes and compares the initial and final scores in all cases during the period of hospital admission. Patients' scores on discharge are generally less than on admission, especially for activity scores.

Conclusion

There is clearly a need to be able to document outcome of RA in the routine clinical setting. This could be done using a physician global assessment or the OSRA. In the clinical trial setting the statistically generated disease activity index may be preferable. In order to make valid comparisons it is important to establish that patient characteristics in the centres are the same. If most of the patients in one clinic have early disease and most of those in another clinic have late disease the use of drugs and resources will inevitably be different. Before conducting an audit it is important to make sure we are not comparing apples and oranges. The OSRA therefore describes the patients in terms of their age, gender and disease duration and is suitable for use in routine clinical practice.

APPENDIX: OSRA scoring system

A *Current disease activity*	0	1	2
1. Well-being. The patient is asked how he feels compared to his last visit.	Same or better	Worse	Much worse
2. Pain. The patient is asked to describe his pain in the last week.	Mild	Moderate	Severe
3. EMS. The patient is asked how long he was stiff for that morning.	< 30 minutes	30–60 minutes	> 60
4. Active joints. The following joints are examined: shoulders, elbows, wrists, MCPs, PIPs, hips, knees, ankles, MTPs. An active joint is swollen ± hot, ± tender. MCPs MTPs, PIP count as one joint.	< 3	3–10	> 10
5. Extra-articular disease.	None	New nodules	Other, eg: vasculitis serositis

B. *Cumulative disease damage*			
1. Function: The patient is asked: (a) Do you get out of the house? (except in other people's cars) (b) Can you dress yourself? (c) Can you feed yourself? (d) Can you climb stairs?	Mild	Problems to: feed, ± dress, ± climb stairs	House-bound
2 Social life: The patient is asked if his social life is as active as that of a healthy person his age.	Normal	Moderately impaired	Severely impaired
3. Number of destroyed or replaced large joints (hips, knees, shoulders).	0	1–2	≥ 3
4. Small joint damage (hands, feet, neck).	Mild	Needs collar, special shoes, hand splints	Surgery done or needed
5. Organ impairment (present for more than 6 months).	None or mild	Skin or muscle	Other organ

11 | Issues of data collection

Roy Carr-Hill
Senior Research Fellow for Medical Statistics,
Centre for Health Economics, University of York

Introduction

An estimated 8 million individuals consult their general practitioner (GP) for rheumatic disorders each year, accounting for some 23% of all consultation with GPs (Dieppe and Paine, 1994). The breakdown of consultations for ICD Chapter XIII (WHO, 1980) (muscular-skeletal disorders) by age and gender according to the data collected in 60 practices for the Fourth National Morbidity Survey of General Practice in 1991 and by the 500 GPs reporting to Inter-Continental Medical Statistics for women aged 20 and over are presented in Table 1. Even from middle ages, at most 13% of all consultations are for Chapter XIII.

Some of these may be relatively minor conditions, although in a recent interview survey 10% of 16–74 year olds reported having

Table 1. Consultations for rheumatoid arthritis for women aged 20 or over

Age group	Total women surveyed	Consultations for any reasons	Consultations for Chapter XIII	Percentage for all consultations for Chapter XIII
20–29	42,746	19,844	7,070	0.037
30–39	37,183	163,259	10,171	0.062
40–49	32,912	139,415	15,018	0.108
50–59	23,683	114,791	14,907	0.130
60–69	22,836	115,851	14,168	0.122
70–79	19,139	106,188	13,941	0.131
80 and over	12,406	68,670	8,011	0.117

Source: Fourth National Morbidity Survey of General Practice, 1991–2 (McCormick *et al*, 1995).

personally suffered from severe arthritis or rheumatism
(HEA/MORI, 1995). Whilst the accepted wisdom is that most
acute rheumatic problems are self-limiting (Dieppe and Paine,
1994), there is little actual evidence. A recent study of shoulder
pain in primary care suggests that, for the majority of patients with
this common problem, disability persisted even 6 months after
presentation.

Rheumatoid arthritis is therefore a substantial problem for purchasers in purchasing for health gain; and practitioners need to
know when to treat, refer or ignore. Efficient methods of collecting reliable data need to be designed in order to be able to
purchase and provide effectively. These 'methods' need to
include a sampling design, choice of 'outcome' measures, and
procedures for data capture. The purpose of this short note is to
document the difficulties in designing such a protocol for this
type of condition.

Measuring outcomes not effects

It is important to underline that we are concerned with the outcomes rather than the effects of any particular 'treatment' for
rheumatoid arthritis. The use of inverted commas is not meant as a
reflection upon the efficacy or otherwise of (any particular) treatment protocol; but, recalling the definition of outcome as being a
change in health status *attributable* to the intervention, the possibility that some of the cases presented for treatment are in fact self-
limiting means that no change attributable to the treatment may
actually have taken place.

This poses a particular problem with this type of condition, as
the patient's health status—which, of course, has to be the basis of
any patient centred outcome measure—is highly variable over
time: indeed, it may vary from week to week. It therefore implies
that there has to be a large sample in order to have any hope of
obtaining a stable estimate of effect. Moreover, as the treatment is
concerned with 'pain relief', there is a subjective assessment which
is very important.

Different perspectives on measuring the outcomes

A wide variety of pathways can be followed by a patient through
the health care system with a chronic condition. In primary care,
this could include—in any order—not only the general practitioner and the practice nurse, but also the occupational therapist, the

physiotherapist, and a range of 'alternatives'; in secondary care, a patient might be seen in general medicine or by a specialist in muscular-skeletal disorders. The sampling 'pool' of those to be 'treated' obviously depends on the point in the pathway at which patients are captured.

Each of these various agents will have a different perspective on the measurement of outcomes, and therefore different requirements for a measurement tool. For example, the general practitioner needs to be able to follow up patients over their registered lifetime with the practice; the hospital clinician would like to be able to trace all those he or she has treated wherever they have come from.

Sampling frame

Given that there are doubts over the likelihood of presentation for different levels of severity, there is a problem of choosing an appropriate sampling frame in order to assess the outcomes of any treatment. For, if even only a small proportion of episodes are self-limiting, then a sampling frame based on those patients presenting (including some who are self-limiting) would provide a biased estimate of the outcome of any particular regimen of care.

This is particularly serious for the hospital clinician who is forced to rely on those who present. Whilst he or she can adopt the randomised control trial approach to compare two treatments among those who present, this will still be a problem if there is differential dropout. Even for a GP with a stable practice population, those with the condition may, at different rates, avoid GPs and/or choose to solicit alternative therapies.

From the point of view of a purchaser, moving to a population base independently of any particular practice also has the advantage that respondents can be asked more easily about self-care or about alternative therapies.

The difficulty then is the choice of a sampling frame for the general population and the effectiveness and specificity of a screening instrument. In terms of a sampling frame, FHSA registers and, to a lesser or more controllable extent, GP registers are known to be inaccurate, but Thatcher's missing million has rendered the electoral register equally suspect. The major alternatives are the Postcode-Address File, which is a file of all addresses in the UK (containing approximately 10% errors), or area-based sampling, where the survey organisation first visits each household in the area to establish a sample.

This procedure is expensive and its efficiency depends on the effectiveness and specificity of the screening instruments.

Outcome measurement

Should outcome measurement focus on pain or on mobility?

Both pain and mobility are important non-commensurable effects of rheumatoid arthritis. There have been rather simple attempts to combine them—for example in the Euroqol[c] instrument—but there is substantial evidence that they do not co-vary. Moreover, reports of detailed analysis of data from surveys using the Nottingham Health Profile and the SF-36 suggest that there are order effects (according to which is asked about first) and also that asking about both together produced different answers than when asked about separately.

Change in health status and referral rates of individual patients/groups of patients

There are potentially a wide range of possible condition-specific impacts such as better symptom control and reduced complications. These could be measured directly or indirectly via the incidence of adverse events. There are also more general impacts on self-perceived health and satisfaction with the care provided. Both types of health outcome are potentially measurable and suitable instruments exist which would be tested in the pilot phase of the study.

It might be also be possible to look at the distribution of referrals to different specialties or the rates for different conditions. In terms of patient care, one possible approach might be to see how many of those who were referred, had expected or had wanted this to happen (at least retrospectively). More promising as a proxy would be the number of repeat visits although the sources of variation here are still largely unexplained. It may also be useful to examine the use of pharmaceuticals for rheumatoid arthritis compared to a population norm either derived from data collected by the Prescription Pricing Authority or by Intercontinental Medical Statistics.

Reliability and validity of data

Two brief points here: how accurate are GP diagnostic data; and how good are self-reports?

GP diagnostic data are likely to be influenced by attitudes of GPs about the self-limiting nature of rheumatoid arthritis.

There have been very few validation studies of self-reports. Some clues can be obtained by looking at the variability of reporting between ethnic minority groups. Thus, the self-reports of arthritis according to the Health Education Authority's Health and Lifestyle Surveys (Table 2) show striking differences from the general population with Bangladeshis rarely mentioning arthritis as a current problem but reporting considerably more past experience. Exactly how these reports should be interpreted in cultural terms ('closeness') to an English lifestyle is a matter for conjecture.

Table 2. Reports of rheumatoid arthritis

	Afro-Caribbean	Bangladeshi	Indian	Pakistani	General population
Mentioned frequently	3	2	4	4	5
Experienced	8	13	8	9	10

Data capture

There are several issues which need to be kept in mind when collecting data: control of data; who are the best interviewers; when should data be collected.

Control of data

In this kind of area, the issue of patient control of the collection and interpretation of data is crucial. Patient definitions of desired outcomes have to be taken seriously in the instruments that are developed.

Who are the best interviewers?

The main choice is between professional interviewers, ex-sufferers and therapists. The experience of fieldwork indicates that they will receive different answers from respondents.

When should data be collected

Given the variability of the condition, it is crucial when data is collected. However, this is a problem mostly when the sampling frame is based on those presenting.

Costs of data collection

Data is not cheap

It has to be emphasised that collecting useful, reliable and valid data is not cheap.

The value of larger data sets

A study/survey should be of a certain size in order to demonstrate a statistically significant difference. The problem with such an argument is that most research requires information on several mediating variables in order to test the theory properly; moreover, where there is more than one competing theory, then information has to be collected in several other sets of variables.

In the simple situation where there is one and only one hypothesis at issue, which can be tested with quantitative data, and where the required level of precision in the answer can be specified, then the classic statistical algorithm on sample size provides a criterion for the minimum sufficiency of data to collect. This procedure can in principle be extended to multiple hypotheses when all the hypotheses can be identified in advance.

Decision analysts (for example, Raiffa, 1970) have proposed formulae based on Bayes Theorem which enable one to assess the added value of new information precisely. But a more important factor is whether or not current views are conducive to accepting the results. If they are, then a small amount of data will be taken as conclusive proof (Stinchcombe, 1968). If not, then much more data is demanded and crucially, alternative hypotheses are proposed to account for the results, which have to be tested in their turn.

Conclusion

Rheumatoid arthritis is a substantial problem for purchasers in purchasing for health gain; and practitioners need to know when to treat, refer or ignore. Efficient methods of collecting reliable data need to be designed in order to be able to purchase and provide effectively. These 'methods' need to include a sampling design, choice of 'outcome' measures, and procedures for data capture. The purpose of this chapter has been to document the difficulties in designing such a protocol for this type of condition.

12 | Conclusions and future developments

Andrew F Long
Project Leader, UK Clearing House on Health Outcomes,
Nuffield Institute for Health, Leeds

and

David L Scott
Reader in Rheumatology, Department of Rheumatology,
King's College Hospital, London

Overview

At the conclusion of the one day conference convened in Leeds in December 1993, in which this monograph has its roots, the multi-disciplinary group of participants recommended (Long and Scott, 1994) that:

- the Modified Health Assessment Questionnaire (MHAQ) be used to provide a record of changes in functional status of the rheumatoid arthritis (RA) patient and to assist decisions on appropriate treatment;
- the patient's perspective be assessed and used as part of the consultation process to influence and/or to decide on the next stage of treatment;
- rheumatology practitioners discuss and agree with commissioning authorities the objectives of RA therapies, taking into account the necessary individual focus of such care.

These three recommendations belie the complexity and challenges that any serious debate on the outcomes of routine patient/clinical care, especially the outcomes of a chronic disease such as RA, has to unravel. At its most simple, even if a reliable, valid, sensitive and acceptable measure of outcome can be identified, numerous substantive and practical questions remain to be addressed; for example:

- how often should the data be collected?
- who should collect the data?
- who will pay for its data collection?
- can the data also be collated into an aggregate form as an aid to health care purchasing decision-making?
- and, most challenging of all, can any observed effect be attributed to the health care process itself?

A unifying theme throughout this volume has been the variety of perspectives on outcome. This is summarised in a basic outcomes grid (Fig 1). However, the grid needs to be made more sophisticated to take account of the evolving nature of RA. Thus, different stages of the disease process have different desirable outcomes. As a further step, the core questions in the grid could be extended to embrace the many other methodological and substantive questions (Table 1). The completion of such a three-dimensional grid—for example, for early and late RA—would provide a valuable template to inform the creation of a common data set for exploring the achievement of desired outcomes.

Does measuring outcome make a difference?

Creating a common data set will be expensive. It is thus essential to review whether or not expending effort on collecting outcomes information is worthwhile. Who will use the data on outcome and how?

Defining group	User	Carer	General practice team	Health care commiss- ioner	Hospital team
Reason for interest in outcomes					
Desired outcomes					
Possible outcome measures/ indicators					

Fig 1. The Outcomes Grid: different actors and desired outcomes

Table 1. Key measurement questions

- What measures exist?
- Is the content of the instrument relevant to the particular application/condition?
- Which measures work best—reliable, valid, sensitive and feasible to use within routine practice?
- When should they be administered?
- Over what timescale—short- and long-term?
- Are they acceptable to the patient group and clinicians?
- Do they provide useful information for (clinical) decision-making?
- Are they easy to interpret?
- Do they explore the user's perspective?

Within research, the purpose of collecting outcomes data is self-evident—as a measure of effect, providing an objective indicator of which treatment works (relatively) more or less. Provided the study is designed appropriately, the issue of attribution should also be straightforward. Within routine clinical practice and especially for a chronic disease, the purpose is, however, less clear; at a minimum it is multi-faceted.

At the level of individual patient care, outcome measurement is concerned with monitoring the desired and achieved outcomes (for example, general functioning or quality of life) or monitoring changes in the patient's ill-health (for example, joint damage). Outcome data will form both an end-point (comparison with the patient's ill-health at a previous time point) and a baseline for future outcome measurement. Its use then lies in monitoring the management of the disease and to assist in deciding and informing the next phase of treatment. However, it is fundamental that collecting data on health status does not add to the data collection burden of the practitioner and to ensure that the data collection helps the patient–clinician interaction.

Exploring outcome within a chronic disease is a dynamic not a once only process; outcome measurement involves an ongoing process of monitoring and evaluating the way the disease is developing and the impact of treatment(s). The 'outcome' is, however, not just one single entity. Many indicators may be used, covering both measures of impairment, disability and handicap. This does, however, raise further questions about how the clinician and patient should interpret the data, which measures should have priority, and which should inform the next stage of the individual's treatment.

At the broader aggregate population level, the argument as to whether collecting outcomes data will make a difference is unproven, though common rhetoric. It may be possible to make use of the same outcomes data collected by the clinician suitably modified, for example changes in HAQ scores per unit of resource. This could then be used to monitor the activity and performance of the rheumatology unit over time, as a means of securing funds within the health care trust, and/or for the trust with prospective purchasers. However, great care would need to be taken to ensure that case mix variables were taken into account in the interpretation of such data.

Purchasing for outcomes in the context of a chronic disease such as RA is by no means a straightforward issue, most particularly, questions of attribution, timescale and perspective. Assuring good processes and quality of care are provided is likely to be as, if not more, appropriate; for example, early access to specialist services once RA is confirmed, direct access upon a flare-up and quality care.

How should outcomes be measured?

A number of key issues should be emphasised in exploring health care outcomes (Table 2). Clear, realistic and measurable objectives for the treatment(s), package of care and/or intervention(s) must be drawn up. Both the user and the multidisciplinary team's perspectives on desired outcomes need to be identified. The user's perspective should be incorporated—not just in the form of asking for their assessments but also through identifying user specified

Table 2. Key issues in assessing outcomes

- Establish clear, realistic and measurable objectives for the treatment(s), package of care and/or intervention(s)
- Identify and explore the user's and the multidisciplinary team's perspective on desired outcomes
- Provide a detailed description of the process of care, together with characteristics of the setting and available resources for delivering the care
- Assess both short- and long(er)- term outcomes
- Use measures that are reliable, valid, responsive to change and clinically useful
- Use outcome measures that inform the clinical interaction with the patient

---

expectations and their achievement at this particular point in disease process. That is, the measures used must relate to key dimensions of outcome for the user. Furthermore, given the range of health practitioners involved in care, it is essential to explore their individual contributions (given current pressures for evidence-based practice). At the same time, particularly from the patient's perspective, the multidisciplinary outcome must be assessed. No single measure does this. The (extent of) achievement of agreed patient-centred goals would provide a common denominator and a meeting point for clinical and patient outcomes.

In order to understand the outcome, it is essential that there is a detailed description of the process of care provided, together with characteristics of the setting and available resources for providing the care, in order to explore whether or not this outcome is indeed a possible end result of the process under review. Moreover, both short- and longer-term outcomes must be assessed. Finally, while the selected outcome measures need to be reliable, valid, responsive to change and clinically useful, in order to enhance the probability of monitoring health outcomes, potential outcome measures should help to inform the clinical interaction with the patient, to identify what to do next and to provide a summary (outcome) of what has been successfully achieved so far. The measurement process itself may thus become incorporated into the clinical consultation and treatment review process. At the same time, other measures of the quality of and satisfaction with the service may also need to be collected.

Clinical and service questions

There is a primary need to review and synthesise current information about rheumatoid outcome. When patients are first seen prognostic markers should allow the severity and likely outcome of rheumatoid arthritis to be determined. Those with severe rheumatoid arthritis would then receive maximal therapy with specific anti-rheumatic drugs. The effectiveness of therapy would be judged by resolution of the clinical and laboratory indicators of the disease and the halting of radiological progression and functional deterioration of the disease.

This view does not reflect the present situation. Prognostic markers do not adequately define the disease and predict its outcome in all cases. Treatment often fails to halt progress of the disease, even though the particular therapy has been demonstrated to be effective in randomised controlled trials. Finally, the measurement of disease progression and its outcome remain inexact, and may emphasise clinical as opposed to patient outcome. Joint radiology has its place but is not always clinically relevant, functional assessments are useful but often far removed from the patients' wishes or needs, and quality of life though difficult to quantify is rarely assessed.

National guidelines recommend rheumatoid arthritis is treated in specialist units by rheumatologists and allied health professionals. The individual components for the management of the disease shown to be beneficial in prospective randomised trials include: non-steroidal anti-inflammatory drugs, slow-acting drugs (for example, gold) and corticosteroids, occupational therapy and physiotherapy, certain surgical procedures such as joint replacement of hips and knees, and hospital admission. Most of these approaches are advantageous over 6–12 months. But the paradox remains of short-term gain but long-term disability. There is also far more information about the effectiveness of drug therapy than physiotherapy and occupational therapy.

There are several areas of therapeutic controversy which need examining in further studies. A major instance is the early use of slow-acting anti-rheumatoid drugs, where 'early' means within the first year of the onset of symptoms, or even within 3–6 months of the onset of rheumatoid arthritis. Current evidence (Kirwan *et al*, 1995) suggests that the early use of second line drugs improves function, a finding which is being picked up within routine clinical practice, patients being started on second line drugs at an earlier stage in the course of their disease. Its long-term impact remains to be confirmed. Another area is the use of several second line drugs together. Combination therapy with relatively small doses of several agents, shown to be effective in controlled trials when used alone, can produce sustained and marked therapeutic control (Tugwell *et al*, 1995). As in the treatment of malignancy or tuberculosis, the use of potent drugs in combination may prevent or delay the clonal expansion of resistant cells. If this is indeed the case in the treatment of rheumatoid arthritis, then consideration should be given to the routine use of drug combinations. It is conceivable that clinicians do patients a disservice by using potentially valuable drugs sequentially rather than in tandem.

More broadly, questions which need answering within the next 5 years include:

- does early therapy with slow-acting drugs improve long term outcome?

- should combinations of slow-acting drugs be used?
- what is the effect of physiotherapy, occupational therapy, and patient educational programmes?
- which patients benefit most from surgical intervention?

Such questions need to be answered in both randomised controlled trials and prospective studies undertaken in routine clinical practice.

There is also a more general issue about health service delivery. Traditional research into disease mechanisms, epidemiology and clinical trials must be supplemented by research into how an optimal clinical rheumatology service can improve disease outcome. This requires a national collaborative strategy to optimise successful research in this area and avoid unnecessary reduplication of effort. There is a need to:

- identify optimal outcome measures;
- define the minimum data set to be collected;
- show the extent of variation in clinical practice;
- explore reasons for such variation;
- determine methods to sample outcomes different units; and,
- evaluate information technology needed to collect and collate data.

There are several data sets from rheumatoid patients which have already been collected and can be used for preliminary work. These include the Early Rheumatoid Arthritis Study (ERAS) and (Young *et al*, 1994) the Norfolk Arthritis Register (NOAR) (Symmons *et al*, 1994). Both look at early disease for patients with established disease at several UK hospitals and use a prospective observation study design. There are also ongoing studies of drug therapy, physiotherapy and occupational therapy in North and South Thames regions.

The costs of providing multidisciplinary care for rheumatoid arthritis are high (over £50 million annually); these are likely to rise steeply when new therapies based on biotechnology become available. The costs for the community are also large. Optimising specialist care is essential. Defining the value of multidisciplinary treatment is essential in order to maximise treatment, to ensure value for money and to enable patients to obtain the best possible care.

Closing comments

Current clinical practice and newly introduced interventions need to be appraised through clinical audit. Current practice should be compared with the synthesis of the current research evidence on what works, when and with whom. This leads on to identify ways to modify and improve existing practice. When evidence on effectiveness is lacking, and this is true for much of conventional clinical practice, further research is indicated. Data on desired and achieved outcomes, including patient expectations, must be collected, allowing the monitoring and auditing of the services provided. The emphasis ought to lie on 'doing it the best way' given available resources and the current state of knowledge—what can be expected 'on the average'. The underlying theme is to enhance the quality of health care provided to users.

Assessing outcomes is a challenging task for both the practitioner and the purchaser. This is particularly so with a chronic disease such as RA, with multiple stages, variable course and inexorable progressive deterioration. The range of different interest groups— patient, carer, primary caregiver, specialist, other members of the clinical team, health care commissioner, policy-maker, and researcher—must not be ignored nor subsumed into a simple focus on one to the exclusion of the others. A long-term commitment to evaluation as part of the routine provision of services is required with the underlying aim of both outcomes assessment and provision of better patient care.

References

Affleck JW, Aitken RCB, Hunter JAA *et al.* Rehabilitation status: A measure of medicosocial dysfunction. *Lancet* 1988; **i**: 230–3.

Ahlem M, Sullivan M, Bjelle A. Team versus non-team outpatient care in rheumatoid arthritis. *Arthritis Rheum* 1988; **31**: 471–9.

Alarcon GS, Lopez-Mendez A, Walter J *et al.* Radiographic evidence of disease progression in methotrexate treated and nonmethotrexate disease modifying antirheumatic drug treated rheumatoid arthritis patients: a meta-analysis. *J Rheumatol* 1992; **19** (12): 1868–73.

Amor B, Herson D, Cherot A *et al.* Follow-up study of patients with rheumatoid arthritis over a period of more than 10 years (1966–1978): analysis of disease progression and treatment in 100 cases. *Ann Med Intern* 1981; **132**: 168–73.

Amos RS, Constable TJ, Crockson AP *et al.* Rheumatoid arthritis: relation of serum C-reactive protein and erythrocyte sedimentation rates to radiographic changes. *Br Med J* 1977; **i**: 195–7.

Anderson J, Firschein H, Meenan R. Sensitivity of a health status measure to short-term clinical changes in arthritis. *Arthritis Rheum* 1989; **32**: 844–50.

Arend WP, Dayer JM. Cutokines and cytokine inhibitors or antagonists in rheumatoid arthritis. *Arthritis Rheum* 1990; **33**: 305–15.

Arthritis Care. *Primary health care for people with arthritis.* Quality Guidelines No. 1, London: Arthritis Care, 1992.

Arthritis Care. *Secondary health care for people with arthritis.* Quality Guidelines No. 2, London: Arthritis Care, 1994a.

Arthritis Care. *Community health care for people with arthritis.* Quality Guidelines No. 3, London: Arthritis Care, 1994b.

Balaban D, Sagi P, Goldfarb N *et al.* Weights for scoring the quality of well-being instrument among rheumatoid arthritics: a comparison to general population weights. *Med Care* 1986; **24**: 973–80.

Berzon RA, Simeon GP, Simpson RL *et al.* Quality of life bibliographies and indexes: 1993 update. *Quality of Life Research* 1995; **4**: 53–73.

Bindman A, Keane D, Lurie N. Measuring health changes among severely ill patients. *Med Care* 1990; **28**: 1142–52.

Bishop D, Green A, Cantor S *et al.* Depression, anxiety and rheumatoid arthritis activity. *Clin Exp Rheumatol* 1987; **5**: 147–50.

Bombardier C, Ware J, Russell I *et al.* Auranofin therapy and quality of life in patients with rheumatoid arthritis: results of a multicentre trial. *Am J Med* 1986; **81**: 565–78.

Bombardier C, Rabout J, Auranofin Cooperating Group. A comparison of health-related quality of life measures for rheumatoid arthritis research. *Control Clin Trials* 1991; **12**: 243S–56S.

Borg G, Allender E, Lund B *et al.* Auranofin improves outcome in early rheumatoid arthritis. Results from a 2-year double blind, placebo controlled study. *J Rheumatol* 1988; **15**: 1747–54.

Bowling A. *Measuring Disease.* Buckingham: Open University Press, 1995.

British Society of Rheumatology. *Musculoskeletal Disorders: Providing for the Patient's Needs. The Role of Rheumatology Departments.* London: British Society of Rheumatology, undated.

British League Against Rheumatism. *Purchasing quality services for people with rheumatic diseases,* 'Purchasers Pack'. British League Against Rheumatism, 1994.

Callahan LF, Brooks, RH, Summey JA *et al.* Quantitative pain assessment for routine care of rheumatoid arthritis patients using a pain scale based on activities of daily living and a visual analog pain scale. *Arthritis Rheum* 1987; **40**: 630–6.

Callahan LF, Pincus T. Formal educational level as a significant marker of clinical status in rheumatoid arthritis. *Arthritis Rheum* 1998; **31**(ii): 346–57.

Capell HA, Porter DR, Madhok R *et al.* Second line (disease modifying) treatment in rheumatoid arthritis: which drug for which patient? *Ann Rheum Dis* 1993; **52**: 423–8.

Carr AJ and Thompson PW. The Disease Repercussion Profile is a valid and reliable measure of patient-perceived handicap in rheumatoid arthritis. *Arthritis Rheum* 1994a; **37**(suppl): S200.

Carr A and Thompson PW. Towards a measure of patient-perceived handicap in rheumatoid arthritis. *Br J Rheumatol* 1994b; **33**: 378–82.

Carr-Hill RA, Dixon P, McIver S. *The NHS and Its Customers: Vol III Customer Feedback Surveys: A Review of Current Practice.* York: University of York, Centre for Health Economics, 1989.

Carr-Hill RA. When is a data set complete: a squirrel with a vacuum cleaner. *Soc Sci Med* 1987; **25,** (6): 753–64.

Carr-Hill RA, Rice N, Roland M. *Determinants of Utilisation of General Medical Services: Report to the Department of Health.* York: Centre for Health Economics, University of York, 1987.

Chambers L, MacDonald L, Tugwell P *et al.* The McMaster Health Index Questionnaire as a measure of quality of life for patients with rheumatoid disease. *J Rheumatol* 1995; **9**: 780–4.

Colvez A, Robine JM. Problems encountered in using the concepts of impairments, disability and handicap in a general health assessment survey of the elderly in Upper Normandy. *Int Rehabil Med* 1986; **8**: 18–22.

Co-operating Clinics Committee of the American Rheumatism Association. A controlled trial of cyclophosphamide in rheumatoid arthritis. *New Engl J Med* 1970; **282**: 883–9.

Co-operating Clinics Committee of the American Rheumatism Association. A controlled trial of gold salt therapy in rheumatoid arthritis. *Arthritis Rheum* 1973; **16**: 353–8.

Corbett M, Dalton S, Young A *et al.* Factors predicting death, survival and functional outcome in a prospective study of early rheumatoid disease over fifteen years (1993). *Br J Rheumatol* 1993; **32**: 717–23.

Corvetta A, Giovagnoni A, Baldelli S *et al.* MR imaging of rheumatoid hand lesions: comparison with conventional radiology in 31 patients. *Clin Exp Rheumatol* 1992; **10**: 217–22.

Cuchacovich M, Couret M, Peray P *et al.* Precision of the Larsen and the Sharp methods of assessing radiologic changes in patients with rheumatoid arthritis. *Arthritis Rheum* 1992; **35**: 736–9.

Dacre JE, Buckland-Wright JC. Radiological measures of outcome. *Clin Rheumatol (International Practice and Research)* 1992; **6**: 39–68.

Davis MJ, Dawes PT, Fowler PD. Comparison and evaluation of a disease activity index for use inpatients with rheumatoid arthritis. *Br J Rheumatol* 1990; **29**: 111–5.

Dawes PT, Fowler PD, Clarke S *et al.* Rheumatoid arthritis: treatment which controls the C-reactive protein and erythrocyte sedimentation rate reduces radiological progression. *Br J Rheumatol* 1986; **25**: 44–9.

Dayer JM. Cytokines and cytokine inhibitors or antagonists in rheumatoid arthritis. *Arthritis Rheum* 1990; **33**: 305–15.

de Haas WHD, de Boer W, Griffioen F. Rheumatoid arthritis of the robust reaction type. *Ann Rheum Dis* 1974; **33**: 81–5.

de Kleijn-de Vrankrijker MW. Application of the ICIDH in interview surveys. *Int Rehabil Med* 1986; **8**: 23–5.

Deal CL, Meenan RF, Goldenberg DL *et al.* The clinical features of elderly-onset rheumatoid arthritis. *Arthritis Rheum* 1985; **28**: 987–94.

Department of Health. *The Health of the Nation.* London: HMSO, 1992.

Deyo R, Inui T, Leininger J *et al.* Physical and psychosocial function in rheumatoid arthritis: clinical use of a self-administered health status instrument. *Arch Intern Med* 1982; **142**: 879–82.

Dieppe P, Paine T. Referral guidelines for general practitioners—which patients with limb joint arthritis should be sent to a rheumatoligist? *Reports on Rheumatic Diseases* 1994, Series 3: 1.

Dixon P, Heaton J, Long AF *et al.* Reviewing and applying the SF-36. *Outcomes Briefing* 1994; **4**: 2–26.

Duthie JJR, Brown PE, Truelove LH *et al.* Course and prognosis in rheumatoid arthritis: a further report. *Ann Rheum Dis* 1964; **23**: 193–202.

Edmonds JP, Scott DL, Furst DE *et al.* Anti-rheumatic drugs: a proposed new classification. *Arthritis Rheum* 1993a; **36**: 336–9.

Edmonds JP, Scott DL, Furst DE *et al.* New classification of anti-rheumatic drugs: the evolution of a concept. *J Rheumatol* 1993b; **20**: 585–7.

Ellis RM. Back pain: emphasise activity and support it with services geared to active management. *Br J Rheumatol* 1995; **310**: 1220.

Emery P, Bradley H, Arthur V *et al.* Genetic factors influencing the outcome of early arthritis; the role of sulphoxidation status. *Br J Rheumatol* 1992; **31**: 449–51.

Epstein WV, Henke CJ, Yelin EH *et al.* Effect of parenterally administered gold therapy on the course of adult rheumatoid arthritis. *Ann Intern Med* 1991; **114**: 437–44.

Felson DT. Choosing a core set of disease activity measures for rheumatoid arthritis clinical trials. *J Rheumatol* 1993; **20**(3): 531–4.

Felson DT, Anderson JJ, Meenan RF. Use of short-term efficacy/toxicity tradeoffs to select second-line drugs in rheumatoid arthritis. A meta-analysis of published clinical trials. *Arthritis Rheum* 1992; **35**(10): 1117–25.

Felson DT, Andersen JJ, Boers M *et al.* The American College of Rheumatology preliminary core set of disease activity measures for rheumatoid arthritis clinical trials. *Arthritis Rheum* 1993; **36**: 729–40.

Fifield J, Reisine ST, Grady K. Work disability and the experience of pain and depression in rheumatoid arthritis. *Soc Sci Med* 1991; **33**: 579–85.

Finnstam J, Grimby G, Nelson G. Evaluation of community-based rehabilitation in Punjab, Pakistan I: Use of the WHO Manual, Training Disabled People in the Community. *Int Disabil Stud* 1988; **10**: 54–8.

Fitzpatrick R. The measurement of health status and quality of life in rheumatological diseases. In: S. Newman and M. Shipley (eds) *Psychological Aspects of Rheumatic Disease.* London: Baillière's Clinical Rheumatology, 1993.

Fitzpatrick R, Newman S, Lamb R *et al.* A comparison of measures of health status in rheumatoid arthritis. *Br J Rheumatol* 1989; **28**: 210–6.

Fitzpatrick R, Ziebland S, Jenkinson C *et al.* The social dimension of health status measures in rheumatoid arthritis. *Int Disabil Stud* 1991; **13**: 34–7.

Fitzpatrick R, Fletcher A, Gore S *et al.* Quality of life measures in health care: 1. Applications and issues in assessment. *Br Med J* 1992; **305**: 1074–7.

Fitzpatrick R, Ziebland S, Jenkinson C *et al.* A comparison of the sensitivity to change of several health status instruments in rheumatoid arthritis. *J Rheumatol* 1993a; **20**: 429–36.

Fitzpatrick R, Ziebland S, Jenkinson C *et al.* Transition questions to assess outcomes in rheumatoid arthritis. *Br J Rheumatol* 1993b; **32**: 807–11.

Frank FG, Beck NC, Parker JC *et al.* Depression in rheumatoid arthritis. *J Rheumatol* 1988; **15**: 920–5.

Fries JF. Ageing, natural death and the compression of mortality. *New Engl J Med* 1980; **303**: 130–5.

Fries J, Spitz P, Young D. The dimensions of health outcomes: the Health Assessment Questionnaire disability and pain scales. *J Rheumatol* 1982; **9**: 789–93.

Fuchs HA. The use of the disease activity score in the analysis of clinical trials in rheumatoid arthritis. *J Rheumatol* 1993; **20** (11): 1863–6.

Fuchs HA, Pincus T. Reduced joint counts in controlled clinical trials in rheumatoid arthritis. *Arthritis Rheum* 1994, **37**: 470–5.

Gabriel SE, Luthra HS. Rheumatoid arthritis: can the long-term outcome be altered? *Mayo Clin Proc* 1988; **63:** 58–68.

Gardiner P, Sykes H, Hassey G *et al.* An evaluation of the Health Assessment Questionnaire in long term longitudinal follow up of disability in rheumatoid arthritis. *Br J Rheumatol* 1993, **32**: 724–8.

Gotzsche PC. Meta-analysis of NSAIDs: contribution of drugs, doses, trial designs, and meta-analytic techniques. *Scand J Rheumatol* 1993; **22**(6): 255–60.

Grimby G, Finnstam J, Jette A. In the application of the WHO handicap classification in rehabilitation. *Scand J Rehab Med* 1988; **20**: 93–4.

Grindulis KA, Scott DL, Struthers GR. The assessment of radiological changes in the hands and wrists in rheumatoid arthritis. *Rheumatol Internat* 1983, **3**: 39–42.

Guccione A, Jette A. Multi-dimensional assessment of functional limitations in patients with arthritis. *Arthritis Care* 1990; **3**: 44–52.

Guillemin F, Briancon S, Pourel J. Functional disability in rheumatoid arthritis: two different models in early and established disease. *J Rheumatol* 1992; **19**: 366–9.

Hall R, Warburton A. Finding the published literature. *Outcomes Briefing* 1993; **3**: 3–5.

Harwood RH, Gompertz P, Ebrahim S. Handicap one year after a stroke: validity of a new scale. *J Neurol Neurosurg Psychiatry* 1995; **57**: 825–9.

Hassell AB, Davis MJ, Fowler PD *et al.* The relationship between serial measures of disease activity and outcome in rheumatoid arthritis. *Q J Med* 1993; **86**: 601–7.

Helewa A, Goldsmith C, Smythe H. Independent measurement of functional capacity in rheumatoid arthritis. *J Rheumatol* 1982; **9**: 794–7.

Herbert R, Carrier R, Bilodeau A. The functional autonomy measurement system (SMAF): Description and validaton of an instrument for the measurement of handicaps. *Age Ageing* 1988, **17**: 293–302.

Hess EV, Luggen ME. Remodelling the pyramid—a concept whose time has not yet come. *J Rheumatol* 1989; **16**: 1175–6.

Hopkins A, Scott DL on behalf of the British Society for Rheumatology and the Research Unit of the Royal College of Physicians. Guidelines and audit measures for the specialist supervision of patients with rheumatoid arthritis. *J R Coll Physicians London* 1992; **26**: 76–82.

Hunfeld G. Use of the ICIDH in registration schemes for social security purposes. *Int Rehabil Med* 1986; **8**: 30–1.

Hunneyball I M, Crossley MJ, Crawford A. Pharmacological manipulation of interleukin 1 production and action and its consequences for the control of connective tissue damage. In Glauert AM (ed): *The Control of Tissue Damage.* Cambridge: Elsevier 1988, 165–78.

Hunt S, McEwen J, McKenna S. Measuring health status: a new tool for clinicians and epidemiologists. *J Royal Coll Gen Pract* 1985; **35**: 185–8.

Hunter T, Duncan S, Dew G *et al.* The effects of anti-rheumatic drugs on the production of collagenase and tissue inhibitor of metallopro- teinasse (TIMP) by stimulated rabbit articular chondrocytes. *J Rheumatol* 1984, **11**: 9–13.

Isomaki HA. An epidemiologically based follow-up study of recent arthri- tis. Incidence, outcome and classification. *Clin Rheumatol* 1987; **6** (suppl 2): 53–9.

Jeffreys M, Hyman M, Millard JB *et al.* A set of tests for measuring motor impairment in prevalence studies. *J Chron Dis* 1969; **22**: 303–19.

Jette A, Davies A, Cleary P *et al.* The Functional Status Questionnaire; reli- ability, and validity when used in primary care. *J Gen Intern Med* 1986; **1**: 143–9.

Johansen A, Doyle DV. Age, health perception and rheumatoid arthritis. *Br J Rheumatology* 1993; **32** (Suppl 2): 58.

Jones R, Crutchley Z. *SHIP's Log.* London: Arthritis Care, undated.

Kaarela K. Prognostic factors and diagnostic criteria in early rheumatoid arthritis. *Scand J Rheumatol Supplement* 1985; **57**: 1–54.

Katz J, Larson M, Phillips C *et al.* Comparative measurement sensitivity of short and longer health status instruments. *Med Care* 1992; **30**: 917–23.

Kazis LE, Meenan RF, Anderson JJ. Pain in the rheumatic diseases: investi- gation of a key health status component. *Arthritis Rheum* 1983; **26**: 1017–22.

Kazis L, Callahan L, Meenan R *et al.* Health status reports in the care of patients with rheumatoid arthritis. *J Clin Epidemiol* 1990; **43**: 1243–53.

Kirwan JR. Arthritis and Rheumatism Council Low-Dose Glucocorticoid Study Group. The effect of glucocorticoids on joint destruction in rheumatoid arthritis. *New Eng J Med* 1995; **33**: 142–6.

Krane SM, Amento EP, Goldring MB *et al.* Modulation of matrix synthesis and degradation in joint inflammation. In Glauert AM (ed): *The Control of Tissue Damage.* Cambridge: Elsevier 1989, 179–95.

Kremer JM, Phelps CT. Long-term prospective study of the use of methotrexate in the treatment of rheumatoid arthritis. Update after a mean of 90 months. *Arthritis Rheum* 1992; **35** (2): 138–45.

Lankhorst GJ, Hoppener MGWC, van der Kaaji JE. Preliminary experiences with WHO's ICIDH: a user's report. *Int Rehabil Med* 1985; **7**: 70–2.

Last PM. First experiences with the ICIDH in Australia's largest nursing home. *Int Rehabil Med* 1985; **7**: 63–6.

Larsen A, Dale K, Eek M. Radiographic evaluation of rheumatoid arthritis and related conditions by standard reference films. *Acta Radiol (Diagn)* 1977; **18**: 481–91.

Lee P, Jasani M, Dick W *et al.* Evaluation of a functional index in rheumatoid arthritis. *Scand J Rheumatol* 1973; **2**: 71–7.

Lefebvre C. Difficulties in identifying articles in MEDLINE using indexing terms (MeSH): experience based on attempts to identify reports of randomized controlled trials. *IFM Healthcare Newsletter* 1994; **5**: 10–5.

Lehtinen K, Isomaki H. Intramuscular gold therapy is associated with long survival in patients with rheumatoid arthritis. *J Rheumatol* 1991; **18**: 524–9.

Leigh JP, Fries JF. Predictors of disability in a longitudinal sample of patients with rheumatoid arthritis. *Ann Rheum Dis* 1992; **51**: 581–7.

Liang MH, Rogers M, Larson M *et al.* The psychosocial impact of systemic lupus erythematosus and rheumatoid arthritis. *Arthritis Rheum* 1984; **27**: 13–9.

Liang M, Larson M, Cullen K *et al.* Comparative measurement efficiency and sensitivity of five health status instruments for arthritis research. *Arthritis Rheum* 1985; **28**: 542–7.

Liang M, Fossel A, Larson M. Comparisons of five health status instruments for orthopaedic evaluation. *Med Care* 1990; **28**: 632–42.

Long AF. Exploring outcomes in routine clinical practice: a step by step guide. *Outcomes Briefing* 1995; **5**: 4–9.

Long AF, Scott DL. Measuring health status and outcomes in rheumatoid arthritis within routine clinical practice. *Br J Rheumatol* 1994; **33**: 682–5.

Lorig K, Fries JF. *The Arthritis Helpbook: A Tested Self-Management Program for Coping with Arthritis and Fibromyalgia.* Reading, Mass: Addison-Wesley, 1995.

McConkey B, Crockson AP, Crockson RA. The effects of some anti-rheumatic drugs on the acute-phase proteins in rheumatoid arthritis. *Q J Med* 1980; **42**: 785–91.

McCormick A, Fleming D, Charlton J. *Morbidity statistics from general practice. Fourth National Study 1991–1992.* Series MBS No.3, Office of Population Censuses and Surveys, HMSO, London, 1995.

Mallya RAK, Mace BEW. The assessment of disease activity in rheumatoid patients using a multivariate analysis. *Rheumatol Rehabil* 1981; **20**: 14–7.

Manganelli P, Triose Rioda W. Il methotrexate a basse dosi settimanali nell'artrite reumatoide. Rassegna della letteratura (Weekly low-dose methotrexate in rheumatoid arthritis. Review of the literature). *Minerva Med* 1993; **84**: 541–52.

Masi AT. Articular patterns in the early course of rheumatoid arthritis. *Am J Med* 1983; **75**(6A): 16–26.

Masters JC, Cerreto MC, Mendlowitz DR. The role of the family in coping with childhood chronic illness. In: Burish TG, Bradley LA, eds *Coping with Chronic Disease: Research and Applications,* New York: Academic Press, 1983.

Matsubara T, Hirohata K. Suppression of human fibroblast proliferation by D-penicillamine and copper sulfate in vitro. *Arthritis Rheum* 1988; **31**: 964–72.

Meenan RF, Yelin EH, Nevitt M *et al.* The impact of chronic disease. A socio-medical profile of rheumatois arthritis. *Arthritis Rheum* 1981; **24**: 544–9.

Melzack R. The McGill pain questionnaire: major properties and scoring method. *Pain* 1975; **1**: 227–9.

Meenan R, Gertman P, Mason J. Measuring health status in arthritis: the Arthritis Impact Measurement Scales. *Arthritis Rheum* 1980; **23**: 146–52.

Meenan R, Anderson J, Kazis L *et al.* Outcome assessment in clinical trials. *Arthritis Rheum* 1984; **27**: 1344–52.

Minaire P. Le handicap en porte-a-faux. *Prospective et sante* 1983; **26**: 39–46.

Minaire P. Disease illness and health: theoretical models of the disablement process. *Bull of WHO* 1992; **70**: 373–9.

Mitchell DM, Spitz PW, Young DY *et al.* Survival, prognosis and causes of death in rheumatoid arthritis. *Arthritis Rheum* 1986; **29**: 706–14.

Moens HJ, Ament BJ, Feltkamp BW *et al.* Long-term follow up of treatment with D-penicillamine for rheumatoid arthritis: effectivity and toxicity in relation to HLA antigens. *J Rheumatol* 1987; **14**: 1115–9.

MORI Health Research Unit. *Health and Lifestyle Survey 1992/93.* Report to Health Education Authority, 1994.

Mullen P, Laville E, Biddle A *et al.* Efficacy of psycho-educational interventions on pain, depression, and disability with arthritis adults: a meta-analysis. *J Rheumatol* 1987; **14**(Suppl): 33–9.

Murphy D, Docherty AJP. Molecular studies on the connective tissue metalloproteinases and their inhibitor TIMP, In Glauert AM (ed): *The Control of Tissue Damage.* Cambridge: Elsevier 1988; 223–42.

O'Boyle C, McGee H, Hickey A *et al.* Individual quality of life in patients undergoing hip replacement. *Lancet* 1992; **339**: 1088–91.

O'Sullivan JB, Cathcart ES. The prevalence of rheumatoid arthritis. Follow-up evaluation of the effect of criteria on rates in Sudbury, Massachusetts. *Ann Int Med* 1972; **76**(4): 573–7.

Paimela L, Leirisalo-Repo M, Helve T *et al.* The prognostic value of HLA DR4 and B27 antigens in early rheumatoid arthritis. *Scand J Rheumatol* 1993; **22**: 220–4.

Pincus T. The paradox of effective therapies but poor long-term outcomes in rheumatoid arthritis. *Seminars in Arthritis and Rheumatism* 1992; **21**(Suppl): 2–15.

Pincus T. Limitations of randomized clinical trials to recognize possible advantages of combination therapies in rheumatic diseases. *Semin Arthritis Rheum* 1993; **23**(Suppl): 2–10.

Pincus T, Callahan LF. Formal education as a marker for increased mortality and morbidity in rheumatoid arthritis *J Chron Dis* 1985; **38**: 973–84.

Pincus T, Callahan LF, Sale WG *et al.* Severe functional declines, worse disability, and increased mortality in seventy-five rheumatoid arthritis patients studied over nine years. *Arthritis Rheum* 1984; **27**: 864–72.

Pincus T, Callahan LF, Vaughn WE. Questionnaire, walking time and button test measures of functional capacity as predictive markers for mortality in rheumatoid arthritis. *J Rheumatol* 1987; **14**: 240–51.

Pincus T, Callaghan LF. Quantitative measures to assess, monitor and predict morbidity and mortality in rheumatoid arthritis. *Baillière's Clin Rheumatol* 1992; **6**: 161–91.

Pincus T, Summey J, Soraci S *et al.* Assessment of patient satisfaction in activities of daily living using a modified Stanford health assessment questionnaire. *Arthritis Rheum* 1983; **26**: 1346–53.

Potts M, Brandt K. Evidence of the validity of the Arthritis Impact Measurement Scales, *Arthritis Rheum* 1987; **30**: 93–6.

Prevoo ML, van Riel PL, van-'t Hof MA *et al.* Validity and reliability of joint indices. A longitudinal study in patients with recent onset rheumatoid arthritis. *Br J Rheumatol* 1993; **32**: 589–94.

Pullar T, Capell HA. Editorial. *Br J Rheumatol* 1986; **25**: 2–5.

Ragan CH, Farringdon E. The clinical features of rheumatoid arthritis. *JAMA* 1962; **181**: 663–7.

Raiffa H. *Decision analysis: Introductory Lectures on Choices under Uncertainty.* Reading, Mass: Addison-Wesley, 1970.

Rankin J. Cerebral vascular accidents in patients over the age of 60. 2. Prognosis. *Scot Med J* 1957; **2**: 200–15.

Rasker JJ, Cosh JA. The natural history of RA. A fifteen year follow-up study. *Clin Rheumatol* 1984; **3**: 11–20.

Rasker JJ, Cosh JA. The natural history of rheumatoid arthritis over 20 years. Clinical symptoms, radiological signs, treatment, mortality and prognostic significance of early features. *Clin Rheumatol* 1987; **6** (suppl 2): 5–11.

Reilly PA, Elswood J, Calin A. Therapeutic intervention in rheumatoid arthritis: a case-controlled comparison of seronegative and seropositive disease. *Br J Rheumatol* 1988; **27**: 102–5.

Remvig L, Enk C, Bligaard N. Effect of auranofin and sodium aurothiomalate on interleukin 1 production from human monocytes in vitro. *Scand J Rheumatol* 1988; **17**: 255–62.

Richmond BJ, Powers C, Piraino DW *et al.* Diagnostic efficacy of digitized images vs plain films: a study of the joints of the fingers. *Am J Roentgenol* 1992; **158**: 437–41.

Ritchie DM, Boyle JA, McInnes JM *et al.* Clinical studies with an articular index for the assessment of joint tenderness in patients with rheumatoid arthritis. *Q J Med* 1968; **37**: 393–406.

Rochon PA, Fortin PR, Dear KB *et al.* Reporting of age data in clinical trials of arthritis. Deficiencies and solutions. *Arch Intern Med* 1993; **153** (2): 243–8.

Roy CW, Hunter J, Arthurs Y *et al.* Is handicap affected by a hospital-based rehabilitation programme? *Scand J Rehab Med* 1992; **24**: 105–12.

Rudick R, Miller D, Clough J *et al.* Quality of life in multiple sclerosis: comparison with inflammatory bowel disease and rheumatoid arthritis. *Arch Neurol* 1992; **49**: 1237–42.

Schnabel A, Gross WL. Low-dose methotrexate in rheumatic diseases—efficacy, side effects, and risk factors for side effects. *Semin Arthritis Rheumatology* 1994; **23** (5): 310–27.

Scott DL, ed. The course and outcome of rheumatoid arthritis. *Baillière's Clin Rheumatol* 1992; **6**: 1.

Scott DL, Huskisson EC. The course of rheumatoid arthritis. *Baillière's Clin Rheumatol* 1992; **6** (1): 1–21.

Scott DL, Panayi GS, van Riel PLCM. Variations between centres when assessing disease activity. *Clin Rheumatol* 1993; **12**: 37.

Scott DL, Panayi GS, van Riel PLCM *et al.* Disease activity in rheumatoid arthritis: preliminary report of the Consensus Study Group of the European Workshop for Rheumatology Research. *Clin Exp Rheumatol* 1992; **10**: 521–5.

Scott DL, Symmons DPM, Coulton BL *et al.* The long-term outcome of treating rheumatoid arthritis: results after 20 years. *Lancet* 1987; **i**: 1108–11.

Scott DL, Coulton BL, Popert AJ. The long-term progression of joint damage in rheumatoid arthritis. *Ann Rheum Dis* 1986; **45**: 373–8.

Scott DL, Coulton DL, Bacon PA *et al.* Methods of X-ray assessment in rheumatoid arthritis: a re-evaluation. *Br J Rheumatol* 1985a; **24**: 31–9.

Scott DL, Dawes PT, Fowler PD *et al.* Anti-rheumatic drugs and joint damage in rheumatoid arthritis. *Q J Med* 1985b; **54**: 49–59.

Scott DL, Grindulis KA, Struthers GR *et al.* The progression of radiological changes in rheumatoid arthritis. *Ann Rheum Dis* 1984; **43**: 8–17.

Segal R, Mozes E, Yaron M *et al.* The effects of methotrexate on the production and activity of interleukin 1. *Arthritis Rheum* 1989; **32**: 370–7.

Sharp JT, Lidsky MD, Collins LC *et al.* Methods of scoring the progression of radiological changes in rheumatoid arthritis. *Arthritis Rheum* 1971; **14**: 706–20.

Sharp JT, Young DY, Bluhm GB *et al.* How many joints in the hands and wrists should be included in a score of radiologic abnormalities used to assess rheumatoid arthritis? *Arthritis Rheum* 1985; **28**: 1326–35.

Sherrer YS, Bloch DA, Mitchell DM *et al.* The development of disability in rheumatoid arthritis. *Arthritis Rheum* 1986; **29**: 494–500.

Sherrer YS, Block DA, Mitchell DM *et al.* Disability in rheumatoid arthritis: comparison of prognosis factors across three populations. *J Rheumatol* 1987; **14**: 705–9.

Short CL, Bauer W. The course of rheumatoid arthritis in patients receiving simple medical and surgical measures. *New Engl J Med* 1948; **238**: 142–8.

Short CL. Rheumatoid arthritis: types of causes and prognosis. *Med Clin North Am* 1968; **52**: 549–57.

Short CL, Bauer W, Reynolds WE. *Rheumatoid arthritis.* Cambridge, Massachusetts: Harvard University Press, 1957.

Sigler JW, Bluhm GB, Duncan H *et al*. Gold salts in the treatment of rheumatoid arthritis. A double blind study. *Ann Intern Med* 1974; **80**: 21–6.

Silman AJ, Reeback J, Jaraquemada D. HLA-DR4 as a predictor of outcome three years after onset of rheumatoid arthritis. *Rheumatol International* 1986; **6**: 233–5.

Singh G, Fries JF, Williams CA *et al*. Toxicity profiles of disease modifying anti-rheumatic drugs in rheumatoid arthritis. *J Rheumatol* 1991; **18**: 188–94.

Situnayake RD. Can disease modifying drugs influence outcome in rheumatoid arthritis? *Br J Rheumatol* 1988; **27** (suppl 1): 55–65.

Smith R. Patient power. (Editor's Choice). *Br Med J* 13 May 1995; **310**.

Steinbrocker O, Traeger CH, Batterman RC. Therapeutic criteria in rheumatoid arthritis. *JAMA* 1949; **140**: 650–62.

Stinchcombe AL. *Constructing Social Theories*. New York: Harcourt, Brace and World, 1968.

Symmons DPM, Barrett EM, Bankhead CR *et al*. The incidence of rheumatoid arthritis in the United Kingdom: results from the Norfolk Arthritis Register. *Br J Rheumatol* 1994; **33**: 735–9.

Symmons DPM, Hassell AB, Gunatillaka KAN *et al*. Development and preliminary assessment of a simple measure of overall status in rheumatoid arthritis (OSRA) for routine clinical use. *Q J Med* 1995; **88**: 429–37.

Taylor D. A table for the degree of involvement in chronic arthritis. *Can Med Assoc J* 1937; **36**: 608–10.

Thompson PW, Pegley FS. A comparison of disability measured by the Stanford Health Assessment Questionnaire disability scale (HAQ) in male and female rheumatoid outpatients. *Br J Rheumatol* 1991; **30**: 298–300.

Thompson PW, Silman AJ, Kirwan JR *et al*. Articular indices of joint inflammation in rheumatoid arthritis. *Arthritis Rheum* 1987; **30**: 618–23.

Tishler M, Caspi D, Yaron M. Long-term experience with low dose methotrexate in rheumatoid arthritis. *Rheumatol Int* 1993; **13**(3): 103–6.

Tugwell P, Pincus T, Yocum D *et al*. Combination therapy with cyclosporine and methotrexate in severe rheumatoid arthritis. *New Eng J Med* 1995; **333**: 137–41.

Tugwell P, Bombardier C, Buchannan W *et al*. The MACTAR Patient Preference Questionnaire - an individualised functional priority approach for assessing improvement in physical disability in clinical trials in rheumatoid arthritis. *J Rheumatol* 1987; **14**: 446–561.

Tugwell P, Bombardier C, Buchanan W *et al*. Methotrexate in rheumatoid arthritis: impact on quality of life assessed by traditional standard item and individualized patient preference health status questionnaires. *Arch Intern Med* 1990; **150**: 59–62.

van der Heijde DM, van Riel PL, Nuver-Zwart IH *et al*. Effects of hydroxychloroquine and sulphasalazine on progression of joint damage in rheumatoid arthritis. *Lancet* 1989; **i**: 1036–9.

van der Heijde DM, van Leeuwen MA, van Riel PL *et al*. Biannual radiographic assessments of hands and feet in a three year follow up of patients with early rheumatoid arthritis. *Arthritis Rheum* 1992a; **35**: 26–34.

van der Heijde DM, van't Hof MA, van Riel PL *et al.* Validity of single variables and composite indices for measuring disease activity in rheumatoid arthritis. *Ann Rheum Dis* 1992b; **51**: 177–81.

van der Heijde DMFM, van't Hof MA, van Riel PLCM *et al.* Judging disease activity in clinical practice in rheumatoid arthritis: first step in the development of a disease activity score. *Ann Rheum Dis* 1990; **49**: 916–20.

van-Schaardenburg D, Hazes JM, de Boer A *et al.* Outcome of rheumatoid arthritis in relation to age and rheumatoid factor at diagnosis. *J Rheumatol* 1993; **20**(1): 45–52.

van Zeben D, Hazes JM, Zwinderman AH *et al.* Clinical significance of rheumatoid factors in early rheumatoid arthritis: results of a follow up study. *Ann Rheum Dis* 1992; **51**: 1029–35.

van Zeben D, Hazes JM, Zwinderman AH. Factors predicting outcome of ' rheumatoid arthritis: results of a follow-up study. *J Rheumatol* 1993; **20**: 1288–96.

Wade DT. *Measurement in Neurological Rehabilitation.* Oxford: Oxford University Press, 1992.

Ware J. Measuring patients' views: the optimum outcome measure. *Br Med J* 1993; **306**: 1429–30.

Weinberger M, Samsa G, Tierney W *et al.* Generic versus disease-specific health status measures: comparing the Sickness Impact Profile and the Arthritis Measurement Scales. *J Rheumatol* 1992; **19**: 543–6.

Weinblatt ME, Weissman BN, Holdsworth DE *et al.* Long-term prospective study of methotrexate in the treatment of rheumatoid arthritis. 84-month update. *Arthritis Rheum* 1992; **35**: 129–37.

Wells G, Tugwell P. Cyclosporin A in rheumatoid arthritis: overview of efficacy. *Br J Rheumatol* 1993; **32**(Suppl): 51–6.

Wells GA, Tugwell P, Kraag GR *et al.* Minimum important difference between patients with rheumatoid arthritis: the patient's perspective. *J Rheumatol* 1993; **20**: 557–560.

Wilke WS, Sweeney TJ, Calabrese LH. Early, aggressive therapy for rheumatoid arthritis: concerns, descriptions, and estimate of outcome. *Semin Arthritis Rheum* 1993; **23**(Suppl): 26–41.

Wilkin D, Hallam L, Doggett M. *Measures of Need and Outcome for Primary Care.* Oxford: Oxford University Press, 1992.

Wilske KR, Healey LA. Remodelling the pyramid—a concept whose time has come. *J Rheumatol* 1989, **16**: 565–7.

Wolfe F, Cathey MA. The assessment and predication of functional disability in rheumatoid arthritis. *J Rheumatol* 1991; **18**: 1298–306.

Wolfe F, Kleinhekel S, Cathey M *et al.* The clinical value of the Stanford Health Assessment Questionnaire Functional Disability Index in patients with rheumatoid arthritis. *J Rheumatol* 1980; **15**: 1480–8.

Wolfe F, Hawley DJ. Remission in rheumatoid arthritis. *J Rheumatol* 1985; **12**(2): 245–52.

Wolfe F, Hawley DJ, Cathey MA. Termination of slow acting anti-rheumatic therapy in rheumatoid arthritis: a 14 year prospective evaluation of 1017 consecutive starts. *J Rheumatol* 1990; **17**: 994–1002.

Wolfe F, Hawley DJ, Cathey MA. Clinical and health status measures over time: prognosis and outcome assessment in rheumatoid arthritis. *J Rheumatol* 1991; **18**: 1290–7.

Wolfe F, Hawley DJ, Cathey MA. Measurement of gold treatment effect in clinical practice: evidence for effectiveness of intramuscular gold therapy. *J Rheumatol* 1993; **20**: 797–802.

World Health Organisation. *International Classification of Impairments, Disabilities and Handicaps (ICIDH), a manual of classification relating to the consequences of disease.* Geneva: WHO, 1980.

World Health Organisation. Division of Mental Health. *Quality of life assessment: an annotated bibiography.* Geneva, 1994.

Yelin E, Meenan R, Nevitt M. Work disability in rheumatoid arthritis: Effects of disease, social and work factors. *Ann Intern Med* 1980; **93**: 551–6.

Yelin E, Lubeck D, Holman H *et al.* The impact of rheumatoid arthritis and osteoarthritis: The activities of patients with rheumatoid arthritis and osteoarthritis compared to controls. *J Rheumatol* 1987; **14**: 710–7.

Young A, Cox N, Davis P *et al.* Treatment patterns over 2 years in 577 patients with rheumatoid arthritis of recent onset. *Arthritis Rheum* 1994; **37** (suppl): S258.

Ziebland S, Fitzpatrick R, Jenkinson C *et al.* Comparison of two approaches to measuring change in health status in rheumatoid arthritis: the Health Assessment Questionnaire (HAQ) and Modified HAQ. *Ann Rheum Dis* 1992; **51**: 1202–5.